T
Handbook

Dr Elizabeth Farrell
& Ann Westmore

ANNE O'DONOVAN
in association with the
Jean Hailes Menopause Foundation

*Published by
Anne O'Donovan Pty Ltd
56 Claremont Street South Yarra 3141
in association with the
Jean Hailes Menopause Foundation*

*Copyright © Dr Elizabeth Farrell,
Ann Westmore and Anne O'Donovan, 1993*

*This book is copyright. Apart from fair dealing
for the purpose of private study, research, criticism
or review, as permitted under the Copyright Act,
no part may be reproduced by any process
without written permission of the publisher.*

*Edited by Margaret Barrett
Designed by Alison Forbes
Cover design by Lynn Twelftree
Typeset in Bembo by Character Typesetters Pty Ltd
North Sydney
Printed by Australian Print Group Maryborough
Distributed by Penguin Books Australia Ltd*

Cataloguing-in-publication entry

*Farrell, Elizabeth, 1948–
The HRT handbook
Bibliography
Includes index
ISBN 0 908476 63 9
1. Hormone therapy. 2. Menopause – Hormone therapy. I.
Westmore, Ann, 1953– . II. Title. III. Title: Hormone
replacement therapy handbook
615.366*

*This book is not intended for self-prescription of Hormone
Replacement Therapy. We advise women to inform themselves about
HRT and then discuss the matter individually with their doctors.*

CONTENTS

ACKNOWLEDGEMENTS 5
INTRODUCTION 7

1 *The menopause – change and challenge* 11
2 *The A to Z of HRT* 35
3 *The benefits* 66
4 *The risks* 91
5 *You and your sex life* 108
6 *Alternatives to HRT* 120
7 *HRT – why, when, how?* 135
8 *Your choice* 164

HORMONES AND DOSAGES 171
HELPFUL ADDRESSES 177
RESEARCH SOURCES 181
INDEX 185

ACKNOWLEDGEMENTS

*M*ANY WOMEN from different walks of life have contributed to this book by sharing with us their experiences of menopause and hormone therapy. We appreciate their candour and their generosity.

Specialist advisers to whom we wish to express our thanks include Professor Henry Burger, Professor James Brown and Ms Assunta Hunter, and we are also grateful to a group of interested men and women, including some medical practitioners, who provided feedback on the manuscript during its final stages. We would like to thank our families, too, for their support at every stage, and publisher Anne O'Donovan and her staff, together with editor Margaret Barrett and designer Alison Forbes, who made many useful suggestions on the content of the book.

We also wish to recognise the invaluable contribution, over many decades, of the biomedical and social science researchers who have provided the sort of systematic information that can help women who are making the transition through menopause. Such research is nowhere near complete, however, and it is vital that the enthusiasm and resources necessary to pursue research in this area are maintained.

Elizabeth Farrell MB, BS, FRACOG, FRCOG
Ann Westmore BSc

INTRODUCTION

*A*s DAUGHTERS, mothers, wives, employers and employees, women in Australia have built careers, raised families, made houses into homes, created successful business enterprises, and cared for the sick and aged. A generation ago women could expect to face such challenges during an average lifespan of around sixty-five years. Today it is about eighty. By the year 2030 it is projected that women over forty-five will constitute a quarter of the population.

Reflecting on the future and its challenges is likely to provoke mixed feelings in the estimated 90 000 Australian women whose menopause will occur this year, and the million or so women who are now in the forty to fifty age bracket. Australian women at midlife tend to be far more positive about ageing than younger people are, but it is the exceptional woman who has no concerns. These may include anxieties about physical and mental health, children, spouses and ageing parents. There may be a fear of financial insecurity – and also of time for important things running out.

On the other hand many foresee good things during 'life after fifty', including active and rewarding years learning new skills and enjoying novel experiences. There is likely to be more time for reading and reflecting, and for pursuing creative and outdoor interests. There should also be liberation from social and biological pressures, and the opportunity to reap the rewards of previous effort on the homefront and in the workforce. Like the French, mature women may consider that if forty-five is the old age of youth, fifty is the youth of second adulthood — their second chance at life.

Good health is important in making the most of these years after menopause, which are likely to occupy as much as a third of a woman's life. Yet the reality is that age-related health problems frequently sap enjoyment and energy at this time.

One of the most controversial and confusing issues for women in the 1990s is how to safeguard their current and future health and wellbeing. There is heated discussion on the appropriateness of hormone treatments for menopausal symptoms, and for reducing serious long-range health problems common in postmenopausal women, including osteoporosis and diseases of the heart and blood vessels.

The HRT Handbook aims to help you find a path through the jungle of information and misinformation about hormone replacement therapy. Its layout is such that you can easily dip into it and find the answers to your questions. It describes what is known and still unknown about the menopause and its effects on women's health. It deals with the experience of natural and artificial menopause among Australian women, with hormone treatments and prescribing practices, and with alternative approaches, natural therapies and research needs.

The book examines common health problems influenced by HRT. The risk of some of these is reduced, of some increased, and the effect of HRT on others remains uncertain — breast cancer being a case in point. Every woman is unique, and her decision about HRT must be made in consultation with her own medical adviser. If she goes ahead with the therapy, the doctor will suggest the hormone or hormones, the format and the dosage that suit her best.

The book considers ways of assessing the costs and benefits

of HRT, assessments that women can apply with their own circumstances and values in mind. Authoritative sources are quoted, and women themselves also raise their voices, telling their own stories and asking dozens of questions.

Making informed decisions about medical treatment is a priority for the baby boom generation, whose members tend to be better informed on health matters than their mothers and grandmothers were. These younger women will work with their doctors but will insist on partnership in the consultation process, and they have every reason for wanting to maintain quality of life for as long as possible.

Women of every age will appreciate that choosing or rejecting treatment with hormones at and after menopause may be one of the most important health decisions they ever make.

CHAPTER 1

The menopause – change and challenge

*A*T FORTY-TWO, Dale Spender was stunned to be experiencing menopausal symptoms. 'It's like a fever,' the feminist author and academic told her friends when the flushes took over her life. 'I'm so hot, and burning and nauseated, and then so cold and shivering. One minute I want to take all my clothes off, the next I need a coat. It's unremitting, happening several times an hour.' Restaurants were out of the question, sleepless nights a frequent occurrence. Work was impossible, and there were so many things she couldn't remember that she thought she had senile dementia. When she complained about the problem, people were generally unsympathetic.

'I thought you would be too busy,' one friend said disappointedly. 'Oh, come on, snap out of it. Find something interesting to do,' said another when she tried to describe how desperate she had become. Always one to put her friends' prejudices to the test, Dale altered her stance. When asked about her health she began to say, 'I'm not very well. I have a fever. Hot and cold flushes. Memory loss. I can't go out anywhere. I can't sleep. It's awful . . . and it's called *malaria*.' Now everyone rushed to comfort her: 'Poor you. Do you have something to take for it?' Friends who had previously advised her to take nothing for her flushes quickly changed their tune.

Eight years later Dale said it still made her angry that the treatment that helped to relieve her 'malaria' was hormone replacement therapy, widely known as HRT. It is not surprising that she was angry. This independent woman had, after all, spent thirty years of her life taking hormone pills, first for contraception and then for menopause.

Before deciding to embark on HRT she gave 'just about everything else' a try, but to no effect. She also had an altercation with one (male) GP who, when asked to explain the mechanics of hot flushes and HRT, said: 'Your thermostat isn't functioning properly and the pill fixes it.' She refused to pay a medical fee for what she considered to be 'electrical appliance' advice and consulted another (female) GP, who admitted that she didn't know why a woman's temperature should rise in these circumstances. In any event the therapy proved successful: the flushes were banished and her life was restored.

Making the decision to go onto HRT was not difficult in the end. 'I think I would have considered suicide eventually, not only because of the relentless symptoms but because of the unsympathetic treatment I got.' The really difficult part was, and is, living with her decision. 'I don't like taking any drugs, including HRT, even though I'm down to the minimal dose. There's also something inside me that's quite perplexed that the flushes and sweats should be part of nature. In so many other areas, if your body is given the right exercise, good food, and is not overstressed, it responds accordingly. The return of symptoms, when I take a break from HRT, makes me feel so powerless. And the fact that I'm still regularly pumping these pills into my body is a source of stress in my life.'

Dale Spender says that if there were any other way, 'even taking an ice-cold bath each day', she'd try it. In the absence of an acceptable alternative, and until she feels strong enough to risk another dose of flushes and sweats, she has decided to continue with HRT.

It was a typical sort of day for Margaret: travelling, making speeches, needing to keep focused, forever in the public eye. She was speaking confidently, in full flow, when suddenly the words stopped. Her mind went blank – as if her brain had seized up or disengaged from everything around about. 'It was like my brain switched off,' she recalled later. 'I couldn't conceal it and tried to laugh it off. But it was very embarrassing and frustrating, on a different scale altogether from ordinary forgetfulness. I hoped that no one realised how bad I felt about it and how frightening it was for me.'

That episode and others like it were among the major reasons why Margaret, then in her mid-fifties and a prominent figure in Australian public life, sought medical help. (Like many other women whose stories are told in this book, Margaret prefers not to use her real name; in her case it is because many of the men in her line of business are liable to make her menopausal symptoms the butt of their feeble jokes.) At about the same time as her memory lapses occurred, she was having hot flushes day and night. She would wake feeling wet along the folds of her skin. Before sleep had a chance to return, her mind would swing into action with details of the busy days ahead. For about six to eight months she also experienced painful abdominal cramps similar to those she remembered from her adolescence; her periods at this time were irregular and sometimes heavy.

Given her frantic lifestyle, the bleeding was quite worrisome. 'I never knew when my period was going to arrive. It was hard to be prepared, and I felt it was all getting too difficult to handle.' The first doctor Margaret consulted recommended HRT, but seemed hesitant about the options when she experienced sore breasts and very heavy periods. 'I went back a couple of times to get a different brand or dose. All up, I tried about three or four different combinations.'

After attending a seminar on the menopause she realised that her doctor was not well informed, and decided to try another medical practitioner. 'She put me onto a patch, which gave me no bothersome side effects except a rash. I changed the position regularly, but eventually I had to give the patch away because I had rash marks all over my buttocks. I was very cross that I was one of the minority of women who experience this reaction.' At the doctor's suggestion she tried several non-drug techniques, including vitamins E and B and evening primrose oil, and these proved helpful within a matter of weeks. Drinking glasses of water before she went to bed also had a beneficial effect.

Margaret still gets flushes but they are less frequent and less severe than previously, and they seem to coincide with times when she neglects to take her vitamin and herbal tablets for a few days. It pleases her that neither her skin nor her vagina is dry, her periods have stopped, and she has no breast soreness. As for the forgetfulness, it doesn't seem so bad these days. 'I still forget things, but it's not like before. At least the computer screen doesn't go completely blank.'

It happens to every woman, sooner or later. Parenthood you can choose or not. With menopause there is no choice. It happens to women who are nurses, secretaries, politicians, news readers, nuns, teachers, doctors, sales assistants and senior executives, to women who are unemployed and to retirees. It happens to women with young children – the menopause mums who are still breast-feeding when their periods stop – to women who have no children, to women working in the home and from home, to those accustomed to a low-stress existence and to those who have consistently demanded the highest mental and physical performance of themselves. Some wish it would happen quickly so that they can throw away their contraceptives and menstruation paraphernalia. Others regret the sometimes sudden, and perhaps also premature, end to their fertile years.

We've talked about the experience of menopause to countless women, the majority of whom have experienced some

As women experience menopause, their feelings about it seem to become more positive than before

signs of change in their body chemistry – hot flushes, headaches, depression, mood swings, sleeplessness. Some are less concerned about these difficulties than about future health problems caused by a possible inherited high risk of heart disease or cancer. Still others have broken a bone soon after menopause and show early signs of reduced bone density (osteoporosis). The questions they ask vary accordingly. Will HRT settle my symptoms? Will it reduce or increase my risk of future disease? Can it stop my existing medical problems getting worse?

We are the first to admit that the women with whom we have discussed the menopause and HRT do not necessarily represent all women. We certainly do not want to stereotype menopause in an excessively negative way. But it is believed that about three out of four women in countries like Australia experience some physical signs associated with menopause, even though only one in four feels she needs medical help to deal with them. Maybe women who don't seek medical advice consider their symptoms to be unimportant, maybe they have not been told about the kinds of help available, or perhaps they are coping perfectly well regardless.

What all women share, whether or not their voices are to be found in this book, is an inevitable change in the function of their ovaries and an end to menstruation. This landmark event – the last menstrual bleed – is what menopause literally means. As your GP will tell you, you can be sure

The term 'menopause' means not just fluctuating hormones, but also children on the move, and altered responsibilities on the homefront and in the workforce

menopause has occurred only when you have had no menstrual bleed for twelve months. Three or so months without a period are not enough: about one in five women near menopause menstruates again after that.

Raise the issue of menopause at any gathering of women, and it is clear that the term has come to mean more than just the end of monthly bleeds. Menopause has become shorthand for the many changes occurring during the transition from regular periods to no periods at all. It is a quick way of summing up hormones in flux, children leaving home or returning, ailing parents needing help, changing relationships with partners, and altered responsibilities in the workplace. An alternative catch-all term for this time of midlife change is the perimenopause.

The last menstrual period for most Australian women occurs between the ages of forty-eight and fifty-three (and can happen quite normally five or so years earlier or later than this). It is less tied to age, however, than at any time in human history due to developments in surgery and cancer treatment. These medical procedures can result in a woman having an artificial menopause (that is, one caused by removal of or damage to the ovaries) from the age of puberty onwards.

Early menopause

Women can experience menopause in their early forties or before. In some women early menopause occurs because of medical intervention, and is described as artificial menopause. For others there is no intervention – they have a 'natural' menopause. The most common type of artificial menopause, surgical menopause, occurs when a woman's ovaries are removed because they are making other medical conditions worse or these conditions are damaging the ovaries.

Endometriosis is one such condition. The endometrium is the lining of the womb (uterus), shed during the menstrual period, and endometriosis is the presence of endometrial tissue in sites other than the womb. In Valerie's case, endometrial cells passed through her reproductive system to her ovaries, settling on them as well as on other parts in the pelvis and abdominal cavity. There, the endometrial cells multiplied and interfered with the normal function of her ovaries, causing

Valerie's periods to be irregular, prolonged and painful. Intercourse was also painful, and this was not relieved by lubricants or relaxation therapy. She decided to go ahead with surgery to remove the endometriosis. Every effort was made to spare the ovaries, but the extent of the condition meant that this was not possible.

The ovaries may also be removed if they are not functioning normally, because of multiple cysts, for example. The cysts can grow as big as golf balls or footballs or any size in between, damaging other vital tissues in the process. (Surgeons increasingly try to preserve at least part of one ovary if the cysts are not cancerous.)

Then again if, before menopause, you have a hysterectomy in which your ovaries are removed along with your uterus and cervix, you can expect to experience symptoms of menopause within days or months of surgery. About half the hysterectomies carried out in the US are of this comprehensive type (in medispeak, a total hysterectomy plus a bilateral salpingo-oophorectomy). In Australia the figure is believed to be somewhat lower. Losing your ovaries has a lot of bearing on the severity of menopausal symptoms; if they are removed before menopause rather than at or after it, symptoms tend to be more severe.

The more common type of hysterectomy performed in Australia involves removal of only your uterus and cervix, not your ovaries. Somewhat confusingly, this operation is termed a total hysterectomy. In theory, a total hysterectomy should not produce menopause. The only change should be an end to your periods and removal of the problems that made the surgery necessary.

In practice, however, a significant number of hysterectomised women who still have ovaries experience symptoms of menopause up to four years earlier than might be expected.

A possible reason for this is that alterations to the ovarian blood supply occurred during surgery. Another common abdominal operation performed on women, sterilisation by tying or clipping of the fallopian tubes (tubal ligation), does not seem to cause an early menopause.

Recent studies show that approximately one-third of South Australian women and one-quarter of New South Wales women have had a hysterectomy by the age of sixty-five. Included in these figures are a number of women whose ovaries have been removed and who are therefore likely to develop more severe menopausal symptoms than the others.

The most common reason for hysterectomy is irregular, heavy and prolonged bleeding (lasting more than two weeks) that does not respond to treatment. This was the case for Roberta, who was forty-six when her uterus and cervix were removed. On the first occasion of prolonged bleeding she bled for fifteen days on end, after which her doctor recommended a hysteroscopy (a procedure that allows a doctor to view the inside of the uterus by inserting a small magnifying instrument via the vagina and cervix). This investigation did not reveal anything of significance and she was given progestogens (synthetic progesterone), which brought the bleeding to an end.

When a similar thing happened a few years later, a repeat hysteroscopy revealed several fibroids (fibrous growths that start in the muscle layer of the uterus, occur in up to 30 per cent of women, and are a common cause of profuse bleeding). Doctors gave Roberta a choice between putting up with the irregular and heavy bleeding, which they expected would subside after menopause (when fibroids usually shrink), and having a hysterectomy. 'I coped with it for several more months but eventually I couldn't take the bleeding, the lack of energy, and the feelings of uncertainty about when it would end.'

Given that irregular bleeding often occurs in the lead-up to menopause, it comes as no surprise to learn that most of the women in the New South Wales study who had had hysterectomies were aged between thirty-five and forty-nine years, with the highest rate in the forty-five to forty-nine age group.

An artificial menopause can also be caused by chemotherapy, the drug treatment used against many types of cancer. Chemotherapy directed at any part of the body prior to menopause may result in a chemical menopause, but regrettably many women are not warned about this possibility. Marcia was upset to learn while having chemotherapy for leukaemia that her ovaries would no longer function after the treatment. 'It was the last thing on my mind at the time I started chemotherapy, and the hot flushes I experienced some weeks later came as a most unpleasant surprise,' she recalled. 'Fortunately I have three children and wasn't intending to have any more. However, I would have appreciated being told earlier about this effect of chemotherapy.' Menopause may also be caused by radiotherapy to the ovaries, when x-ray treatment is given for a cancer in the pelvis.

Early natural menopause in the absence of any medical intervention is more likely in women who smoke (smokers experience menopause one to two years earlier, on average, than non-smokers and ex-smokers, the reason being that smoking reduces the availability of oestrogen to body tissues). Later menopause is more likely in woman with many children, and women who are heavier than average. Genetic and nutritional factors also seem to play a part: the menopause for Asian women apparently occurs earlier than for those with northern European backgrounds.

Sometimes none of these reasons accounts for spontaneous premature menopause, which on rare occasions can be found in women in their thirties or, even more rarely, in their teens or twenties. Studies suggest that the egg supply of most of these women has run out, but it is not clear whether this is due to a shortage of eggs at birth or, as is more likely, some unknown factor.

Natural menopause

For most women menopause occurs between forty-eight and fifty-three, and it is usually preceded by a few years of changing ovarian function, including an end to the release of eggs (ova). Women may view it as 'one of nature's design faults' or 'a blessed relief from periods and pregnancies'. Each ovary of a newborn baby girl contains about a million immature eggs. Up to five hundred eggs develop to full maturity between puberty and menopause and are released from the ovary in the process of ovulation. No one is sure why the remainder degenerate, nor is it clear what triggers the sex hormone shifts and the stop-starts in ovarian function signalled in the years before menopause by altered bleeding patterns.

About the only certainty is that menopause occurs when the number of eggs in the ovary falls to a critical level.

Menstrual irregularity and contraception at menopause

You may notice your periods becoming irregular in your late forties, although this can occur quite naturally some years earlier or later. As periods become less frequent, your fertility declines. Women of fifty-five have become pregnant, however, and one Californian woman gave birth at the ripe old age of fifty-seven years! The changing output of sex hormones by the ovaries, as the menopause approaches, is responsible for this menstrual irregularity. For most women, irregular periods last between two and seven years, though the range is a few months to eleven years. If you are irregular for many months, this can be a confusing and stressful time because of both the bleeding and the risk of an unplanned pregnancy.

In order to meet contraceptive needs in their forties and fifties, some women use the Pill or long-acting contraceptives like Norplant, a hormone-containing pellet that is implanted under the skin. These tend to mask changes in menstrual bleeding that indicate the approach of menopause.

This was the case for Janet, a Pill-user since having an IUD removed ten years previously. When she was fifty-three and, with no change in her Pill-induced bleeds, experienced a few hot flushes, she asked her doctor if these could be menopause-related. Her doctor recommended that she use a non-hormonal form of contraception for a while to see if her menstrual periods occurred, thus allowing an assessment of what was happening to Janet's own hormone production. After she and her partner had been using condoms for a few months she had a menstrual bleed. She then faced further choices – whether to continue using condoms until her bleeding disappeared for a full year, or to resume the Pill for another year before repeating the same sort of Pill-free 'trial'. Janet chose the first of these options, and what turned out to be her final period occurred four months later. According to a recent Australian study, an increasing number of couples choose sterilisation of one or other partner – at this stage of life another option again.

It is important to point out that the Pill is not a suitable choice for any woman over thirty-five who has a substantial risk of heart and blood vessel disease. Indications of high risk include smoking, high blood pressure, unacceptable blood fat levels, and a family history of heart and blood vessel disease mainly associated with the early death of a relative. If you fall into any of these categories, your risk of suffering a heart attack, a serious blood clot disorder or a stroke markedly increases.

Both HRT and the Pill typically include the hormones oestrogen and progestogen, a synthetic form of progesterone, but the hormone doses in HRT tend to be considerably lower than in low-dose Pills. While women on the Pill who smoke have a measurable increase in their risk of heart disease, the heart health of smokers on HRT does not seem to be jeopardised. In fact, for such women, HRT may confer important health benefits.

Sex hormones produced at and after menopause

Research shows that when the ovaries stop releasing eggs at the menopause, and the lining of the uterus no longer changes in preparation for a possible pregnancy, most women continue to make measurable and useful amounts of active sex hormones. The major source of oestrogen is chemical conversions that take place in fat tissue, hence the amount of body fat has a good bit to do with oestrogen levels in postmenopausal women. The brain and the adrenal glands (two small organs near the kidneys) also continue to produce hormones that control the reproductive system at this stage of your life. Like body weight, your genetic make-up is an important factor in the output of these hormones.

Overall, we produce relatively smaller amounts of oestrogens, progesterone and androgens (a class of hormones that includes testosterone) after menopause than before it, and the balance of the various hormones changes. Testosterone, for example, becomes a more dominant hormone, even though less is produced after menopause than beforehand. The altered hormone balance explains some of the rapid and not-so-rapid changes to the body associated with menopause.

These hormones act on chemical structures called hormone receptors in many parts of the body. Their influence extends to the ovaries, fallopian tubes, uterus, cervix, vagina, vulva, skin, heart, blood vessels, liver, joints, bone, breasts, brain and urethra (the passage from the bladder to the outside). Various forms of oestrogen affect tissues such as the vaginal lining and the blood vessels in quite different ways. For each of us, changes in our hormone balance will be different, and consequently the effects will vary from woman to woman. Thus the increased prominence of testosterone after menopause may cause an increase in facial hair, altered libido (interest in sex), and a change in the distribution of body fat that is quite apparent to some women but goes almost unnoticed by others.

Menopausal symptoms

According to Dr Derek Llewellyn-Jones, a Sydney obstetrician and gynaecologist and a prolific writer on health issues, at least a hundred symptoms have been attributed to the menopause, but only two can be related absolutely to the hormonal changes that are going on. They are hot flushes and vaginal dryness. Nonetheless women in the reproductive years can experience similar symptoms. In any given two-week period, for instance, one in ten women who are not menopausal experiences a hot flush.

Irritability and moodiness are another good example of symptoms not confined to menopausal women, a point made by Dale Spender in the *Sydney Morning Herald* of 14 April 1993. 'Now that we are all familiar with the psychological distress caused by unemployment,' she said, 'we can see that it is very similar to the so-called symptoms of menopausal women. [If they are] Denied a useful role and a sense of affirmation, the outcome is low self-esteem, depression and a sense of futility about the meaning of life. In the past we just confused menopause with "downsizing".' Not only do

SIGNS OF MENOPAUSE

You may become aware that menopause is around the corner when some or all of the following signs show up:
- unpredictable menstrual bleeding that is sometimes very light and regular, at other times heavy and prolonged
- hot flushes and accompanying sweats
- bladder problems resulting in a need to urinate more frequently and troublesome urinary tract infections
- uncharacteristic irritability and mood swings
- short-term memory loss and difficulties with concentration
- sleeplessness and a generalised loss of zip
- a crawling sensation under the skin
- inexplicable weight gain and shifts in body fat distribution
- dryness of the vagina, making intercourse painful or less comfortable
- loss of libido
- less frequent appearance of the lubricative mucus from the cervix that indicates ovulation
- headaches, dizziness, heart palpitations

women of menopausal age sometimes experience feelings of scaled-down worth, they are also coping with the physical effects of fluxing hormones. Perhaps they might handle the situation better if they did not have to cope with these dual pressures simultaneously.

Lasting physical changes

As well as the signs of menopause we have listed, which usually last for several months or years, some longer-term body changes get a hurry-on at around the time of menopause. These may be caused by both the altered output of sex hormones and other physiological and biochemical changes that affect men as well as women. They typically occur over many years and include some or all of the following.

- There is a reduction in bone strength and density that is most pronounced in the first five to six years after menopause. Whether this translates into an increased risk of fractures depends on many things, including the strength of the bones in the first place (that is, the peak bone mass) and the rate at which bones lose density. (Men experience a similar decline in bone density in later life, but not the rapid loss that women have in the first few years after menopause.)
- The strength of the support tissues of the body, such as muscles and cartilage, may also decline. This can lead to backache, joint and muscle pain, and trouble with your 'waterworks' from time to time. A prolapse may also occur if the uterus, bladder or bowel moves down into the vagina because of weakened pelvic muscles and ligaments. Surgery or the insertion of a polythene ring or pessary into the vagina may be necessary to lift the pelvic organs away from the pelvic floor. Occasionally a hysterectomy may be performed to overcome a serious prolapse problem.

- For some women there is a declining desire for sex ('I'd just as soon curl up with a good book'), while for others, one of the redeeming features of menopause is the discovery or rediscovery of their sexuality.
- The blood flow to the sex organs may be reduced, and the nipples and clitoris may become oversensitive.

How long do menopausal problems last?

Studies of large groups of women in Western countries indicate that about 70 per cent experience menopausal problems they regard as moderately distressing. A further 10 per cent of women describe their symptoms as severe, and 20 per cent get through the menopause with barely any disturbance.

In some women the signs of menopause last a few months, in others for two or three years. About a third of women are still experiencing distressing problems five years after their last period, and about a fifth have disturbances including hot flushes for a total of ten years. In general, you will be relieved to know, the severity of symptoms decreases with time.

The place of hormone measurements

Even before your menstrual periods become noticeably irregular, there are subtle changes going on in your ovaries. Studies involving the monitoring of women's sex hormones over many years show that there are small shifts in hormone levels for about ten years before the last menstrual bleed. This contrasts with the view held by many women that menopause is a relatively sudden life change.

Denise, for example, regarded menopause as a swift transition, since she was keenly aware of changes for only a little more than a year. 'I was shocked when my always-predictable menstrual cycle went haywire. Instead of five days, I was bleeding for eight days and my cycle got longer. Then things went back to near-normal for a while, before I had bleeding and spotting for nearly two weeks and another long cycle. This sort of irregularity continued for about fifteen months, including a month when I had nineteen days of bleeding and spotting with just two days relief in the middle. I have a theory that this irregular bleeding helps women adjust to menopause in a positive way. I mean, when I looked back and could see that menopause had occurred, I was truly relieved that my body had become predictable once again.'

By the time symptoms are obvious, sex hormone levels can be fluxing significantly from day to day. Interpretations of hormone measurements at this time are notoriously misleading, which is why most doctors prefer to rely on symptoms as the most useful guide to the stage of menopause. In a

Most women have irregular periods for two to seven years leading up to menopause

world where we rely on tests in so many areas, this may seem unsatisfactory. But the fact is that despite sophisticated hormone measuring systems, there is still no test to show that menopause is occurring or to predict just when the last menstrual bleed will take place.

There are some situations in which hormone tests can be very helpful indicators of what is happening to the reproductive system. These include the following:
- after a woman's own hormone production has stabilised and her menopause is confirmed;
- in women who have had a hysterectomy or an artificial

menopause and are experiencing distressing symptoms; and
- in women who have been given sex hormones in the form of implants (see chapter 2).

Factors influencing menopausal symptoms

The menopause is a time of transition, a nudge that sets us thinking about what is behind us and what we want from the years ahead. Both the internal changes of our bodies and their interaction with other factors in our lives seem to influence the symptoms of menopause that we experience.

HORMONE LEVELS   There is no doubt that problems such as hot flushes and vaginal dryness are associated with the sex hormone changes of the menopause. Hot flushes have been linked with rising levels in a brain hormone called luteinising hormone and falling levels in the most powerful form of oestrogen, oestradiol (see page 172). The changed balance of hormones also helps to explain symptoms of vaginal dryness and urinary frequency. Hormones are not the only controller of symptoms, however.

ANXIETY   Sudden bouts of anxiety seem to be linked with hot flushes in some women. The more anxious you feel, the more likely you are to have hot flushes.

SEXUAL ACTIVITY   Even though vaginal dryness and painful intercourse are often blamed for reduced sexual activity and arousal in women after menopause, it is not clear which is the cause and which the effect. Research suggests that women who don't often have sex tend to have more problems with vaginal dryness than those who have it frequently. In addition, the more often a menopausal woman is sexually aroused and active, the more easily natural vaginal lubrication is achieved, and the more comfortable and enjoyable sex tends to be.

As discussed in chapter 5, the use of vaginal lubricants and 'male dew', or hormone therapy, may break the cycle of discomfort that is sometimes associated with sexual activity, and result in the release of natural lubricants. This is not to suggest that arousal is merely a physical matter; psychological influences to do with mood, touch, words and images are also important. Libido is not merely a matter of hormones. What is in your head and heart will also affect your interest in sex, and such things are not dependent on HRT. Interestingly, sex may have an influence beyond stimulation in preventing genital dryness as, according to research conducted by family planning authority Professor Egon Diczfalusy from the Karolinska Institute in Sweden, semen itself – absorbed through the vaginal walls – is a rich source of oestrogen.

STRESS Extreme demands on physical and mental energy, loosely termed stress, increase the tendency to flush. Hot and stuffy rooms, excessive amounts of alcohol and caffeine, a poor diet, sleep deprivation and thyroid disorders are common stress-related triggers of hot flushes.

Attitudes to menopause

Positive attitudes to menopause and ageing have been linked with fewer menopausal symptoms, as have education and income level, occupational status, cultural background, and dietary and genetic characteristics. Japanese women are often cited as a shining example of a group with positive attitudes to menopause – women who are much less likely to report symptoms such as hot flushes than their middle-aged sisters in the West. To attribute their low incidence of symptoms to their positive views of menopause is an oversimplification, however, since there would appear to be many other contributory factors. For instance, Japanese women tend to have lower oestrogen levels than Western women both before and after menopause (apparently due to dietary and genetic influences), and their hormone level changes may be less acute and therefore less troublesome.

Early results of the Melbourne Women's Midlife Health Study suggest that most women aged forty-five to fifty-five and born in Australia are quite positive about menopause and ageing in general. Most of the 2000 randomly selected women

Problems associated with menopause affect about 70 per cent of Australian women, but only a minority seek medical advice

who were questioned were not worried about being too old to have children. Two-thirds were not concerned about their children leaving home, nor were the majority anxious that their attractiveness was waning. About half thought that some women became depressed or irritable in midlife, but most believed that the transition was hardly noticed by women with many interests. Only 9 per cent of these women rated their health as worse than that of other women of the same age. Over 90 per cent experienced some symptoms of ill health, particularly generalised aches and stiff joints, lack of energy, nervous tension, headaches and migraines. But most women regarded these as relatively minor concerns.

A comparable US study, which followed for five years the wellbeing of more than 2000 middle-aged Massachusetts women selected at random from the general population, came up with interesting findings on the pattern of such symptoms over time. On the one hand, lack of energy, feeling blue or depressed, headaches and menstrual problems were reported much less often at the end of the five years than at the beginning. The reverse was true for hot flushes and cold sweats, which were reported nearly twice as often.

Another intriguing discovery was the shift in attitudes to menopause as experience took over from expectation. At the beginning of the study about 70 per cent of those questioned said they would feel relieved or neutral when their menstrual periods stopped, and 3 per cent expected to feel regretful. Five years later, the overwhelming majority of women were positive or neutral about menopause. In other words, as women experienced menopause, their feelings about it became more positive.

One explanation for this positive shift could be that women have been 'sold' too pessimistic a view of menopause and feel relieved when they successfully negotiate it. The pessimistic sales pitch arises from folklore belonging to past eras and, paradoxically, to scientific studies of women's health, many of which have concentrated solely on users of the health care system. These studies are biased because participants tend to be women experiencing the most difficulty, who do not represent all women.

Another possible explanation for the shift in views could lie in evolving approaches by women to their own health problems. Many women are becoming more aware, more questioning, and they are educating themselves better on health issues than did their mothers and grandmothers. 'We have a growing population of consumers who do not accept drugs or the doctors' say-so any more,' says Nancy Peck, former coordinator of the Healthsharing Women's Health Information Service funded by the Victorian Health Department and the National Women's Health Program. Women like Ms Peck were in their thirties in the 1970s and were vocal about issues like rape, abortion and the Pill. As she enters her fifties, she and other women of her generation are speaking out about key issues such as menopause and HRT.

The current generation of forty-year-olds and fifty-year-olds has benefited also from weakened taboos associated with sex, reproduction, menstruation and menopause. While we are living longer and have more reason to worry about heart disease, fractures, strokes, lung cancer and breast cancer than previous generations of women, we are talking openly about these health problems within the family, and usually with friends and trusted doctors as well, discussing how we might tackle them in our own lives and in the lives of our daughters and grand-daughters.

Differing views of menopause

Modern medicine tends to equate the menopause with a formidable array of symptoms, and longer-term deterioration of body tissues that it blames on oestrogen deficiency. The implication is that menopausal women need hormone therapy to minimise or avoid symptoms and to maintain good health into old age. This view of menopause is increasingly under attack as oversimplified. Critics say that the absence of serious menopausal problems in many women who undoubtedly experience an overall drop in oestrogen (and other sex hormone) levels has not been adequately explained.

Some critics of the medical view also argue that the increased incidence of many diseases attributed to menopause may largely reflect ageing processes that would occur even if there were no such life stage as menopause. Others say that the focus on hormonal factors leads to the neglect of other possible biological contributors to symptom development and later health problems. These include lack of exercise, smoking, and poor nutrition involving inadequate vitamin and mineral intake. There is also criticism of the tendency to neglect psychological and social influences on mood states like irritability, depression and anxiety, which may be glossed over as 'menopause-related' without further investigation. The emergence of these symptoms at menopause may have less to do with hormones than with the reappraisal of personal relationships, or changes in self-confidence or self-esteem.

Although the medical view is widely criticised, women themselves are often the first to vouch for the effectiveness of oestrogen in relieving distressing symptoms like flushes and sweats. There is also good evidence that oestrogen has a beneficial effect on bone structure and blood vessel function, in some women at least. The challenge facing thoughtful doctors and those who run menopause clinics is to try to work out, in conjunction with their patients, the pluses and minuses of hormone use. And it is imperative that women learn all they can, so that they are equipped to make informed decisions in favour of HRT or against it.

CHAPTER 2

The A to Z of HRT

THE EXPERIENCE of menopause is a roller coaster ride for some women, and the history of menopause-related sex hormone therapy has also had its ups and downs. Early this century medical practitioners and alternative therapists used powdered and desiccated concoctions prepared from animal ovaries as remedies for many physical and mental disorders in women. All sorts of problems were blamed on ovarian malfunction, and it seemed logical to look to healthy ovaries for a solution. The preparations given to women were full of impurities, however, and the results were unpredictable and discouraging.

Hormone replacement therapy as we know it today had its beginnings in the late 1920s, when the form of oestrogen now known as oestrone (see page 171) was first isolated from the urine of pregnant women. A later (1943) development was the extraction of an oestrogen from the urine of pregnant mares. This preparation, called conjugated equine oestrogen, was, and continues to be, prescribed widely under the brand name Premarin.

The next big development had nothing to do with science and everything to do with marketing. In 1963 the Wilson Foundation was established in New York by the Brooklyn gynaecologist Dr Robert A. Wilson, and backed by $US1.3 million in grants from the pharmaceutical industry. The foundation's mission was to promote the use of oestrogens and Wilson succeeded in this, particularly through his widely read book *Feminine Forever*. In an article summarising his book, Wilson described menopausal women as 'living decay', and said that oestrogen therapy could save them from being 'condemned to witness the death of their womanhood'. He listed twenty-six symptoms that the 'youth pill' could avert – including hot flushes, osteoporosis, thinning of the vaginal walls, sagging and shrinking breasts, wrinkles, absent-minded episodes, irritability, frigidity (a condition rarely referred to these days!), depression, alcoholism and even suicide.

Women's acceptance of oestrogen was helped along by the statements of medical authorities such as Dr Robert Greenblatt, a leading endocrinologist who was president of the American Geriatrics Society. In 1974 Dr Greenblatt claimed that about three-quarters of menopausal women were acutely oestrogen-deficient, and he advocated oestrogen therapy for them all, even in the absence of symptoms. A year later, with prescriptions for oestrogen exceeding 26 million in the US alone (it was the fifth most frequently prescribed drug), and worldwide sales of Premarin surpassing $US100 million in value, controversy erupted.

Two independent studies by reputable US research teams, both published in the *New England Journal of Medicine* in 1975, reported a link between postmenopausal oestrogen therapy and cancer of the endometrium (the lining of the uterus), the risk increasing with the duration of therapy and its dose. The researchers found that women who had a uterus and used oestrogen preparations without any other sex hormones, such as progestogens (synthetic forms of progesterone), for longer than six months had an increased risk of endometrial cancer – five to ten times greater than was normal for their age.

There followed a period of widespread concern and scientific reappraisal, during which progestogens were teamed with oestrogen, the aim being to protect the endometrium of all women with an intact uterus from the increased risk of endometrial cancer. Subsequent studies have confirmed that progestogen achieves this protection.

Much has been learned from this saga, particularly the need for constant review of present knowledge, and a commitment to ongoing research of the menopause and ageing. What we can say with confidence is that in recent years there has been a resurgence of interest in HRT, together with an acceleration of research and clinical trials using therapies of different dosages in different patient groups, and the development of

> *Adequate doses of oestrogen and progestogen will protect you against cancer of the endometrium if you have a uterus*

new ways to administer it. One of the biggest challenges now facing the medical research community is to identify women who need HRT and those who don't. Women themselves should at the same time be analysing their experience of menopause in the light of their own medical history, weighing up the evidence, and making their own judgement.

Who uses HRT?

Those on HRT are mainly women seeking help to reduce their menopause-related symptoms. In some cases the menopause has occurred naturally. In others menopause has been brought on by removal of or damage to the ovaries during surgery, chemotherapy or radiotherapy (see chapter 1). The main user groups other than women with generalised menopausal symptoms are those who are at high risk of fractures and heart disease, and those already experiencing these health problems.

A study of Massachusetts women aged forty-five to fifty-five found that, of those on HRT after natural menopause, fewer than one-third continued the treatment for more than two years. Among those who had a hysterectomy, nearly two-thirds stayed on hormones for more than two years. Among women in the natural menopause group, those on hormones were different in some important ways from those not on it. Before they started treatment, these women were more likely to have reported hot flushes or menstrual problems than women who did not embark on hormone therapy. They were also more likely to regard their health as poor and to use health services. These women were better educated, too, and were more likely to have used oral contraceptives in the past.

Prescribing HRT for women who do not have clearly defined symptoms and are not at high risk of postmenopausal fractures or heart disease is quite a controversial matter. Fuelling the controversy are some medical specialists who advocate HRT for most women 'from menopause to grave'. Supporters of this approach tend to equate menopause with 'hormone deficiency' or 'ovarian failure', often giving the impression that menopause is a time of dramatic and irreversible shutdown of sex hormone production: the start of a downhill road along which women become crumbling shadows of their former selves. This is a ridiculous generalisation, as the variability in sex hormone production after menopause is vast.

Opponents of the widespread and protracted use of HRT challenge the notion of universal hormone deficiency. They point to big individual differences in sex hormone levels at and after menopause, the difficulty of translating these measurements into symptoms or disease risks, and to the diversity

We need to pinpoint women with special problems at menopause, carefully assess the likely health outcomes with and without HRT, and ensure fair access to tests that can assist decision-making

of experiences of menopause. While conceding that production of oestrogen by the ovaries declines after menopause, they say that older women need less oestrogen. A relatively small amount seems sufficient for the many and varied organs that oestrogen influences.

In most women, oestrogen production by the adrenal glands and by fat and muscle tissue partly compensates for the diminished oestrogen output of the ovaries from menopause onwards. Jill is a woman who found the 'HRT for everyone' approach worrying. Most of her friends seemed to be on HRT, yet at fifty-seven she was in exuberant postmenopausal health without it. For Jill, fitness has been something of an obsession for many years, partly because she has a tendency to put on weight easily: in spite of vigorous daily exercise and a carefully balanced diet she remains 'well covered'. After reassurance that her sensible lifestyle was providing protection for her bones and heart, and her fatty tissue was supplying adequate oestrogen for her needs, she decided that HRT was not necessary for her.

The second main challenge to advocates of near-universal long-term HRT has come from those who question the confidence with which clinicians attribute benefits to HRT that are based on specific research findings. The research quoted usually involves the use of oestrogen on its own, rather than the more usual combination of oestrogen and progestogen (see chapter 4). These critics also argue that, until the results of long-term studies of current HRT formulations and dosages are available, it is foolhardy to widely prescribe hormone therapy without firmer selection criteria than operate at present.

It makes more sense to identify specific groups for whom menopause is a particularly distressing or potentially dangerous experience; to analyse carefully the immediate and future risks and benefits they face, and the pros and cons of HRT in their situation; to upgrade selection criteria; and to campaign for fair access to screening tests that can assist decision-making. This would help to ensure that women in need of HRT have access to it, while those for whom it is unnecessary do not embark on it. Taking up these challenges is, of course, a matter for the women concerned, as well as researchers.

Studies of Australian women aged forty-five to fifty-five indicate that about one in two who have had their ovaries removed at the time of hysterectomy are on HRT, as also are one in three who have had a hysterectomy without removal of their ovaries, and about one in six who have had a natural menopause. In a comparable group of US women, the rate was about the same in the surgical menopause group and significantly lower in the natural menopause group. Rates seem to vary widely across Western Europe, but there are no comparable studies by which to assess this.

What is oestrogen?

There are three main types of oestrogen produced by the body; oestrone, oestradiol and oestriol (see pages 171–2). They influence the functioning of various parts of a woman's body:

- the growth and development of the uterus and its lining (the endometrium)
- the thickness and tone of the vaginal lining and the vagina's production of secretions
- the fullness, tone and secretions of the vulva, cervix and urethra
- bone growth
- temperament and sexual interest, by an action on the brain
- many other body tissues such as the skin, heart, blood vessels, breasts, liver and joints

OESTROGENS USED IN HRT   The main reasons for giving oestrogen at and after menopause are to relieve distressing or debilitating symptoms and to reduce future risk of fractures and heart disease. In general, 'natural' oestrogens are the preferred form of oestrogen in HRT, and a number of alternatives are available (see page 175).

Severe symptoms are especially likely in women who have had a surgical menopause, and this partly accounts for their relatively high use of HRT. They are also more likely to seek treatment than women who have had a natural menopause. Women taking oestrogen alone tend to stay on their hormone therapy for longer than women taking oestrogen plus progestogen (with or without testosterone), perhaps because they do not experience the unwanted side effects sometimes associated with the progestogens.

You may be confused by the distinction made between the 'natural' and the 'synthetic' hormones of HRT. When your doctor describes a particular HRT hormone as natural, this means that it is broken down according to a normal biological pathway of the body. For this to occur, it must have the same structure as a hormone produced by the woman, or a very

> *For any hormone therapy, including HRT, it is prudent to start low and go slow*

similar one. Examples of natural oestrogens include Progynova, Ogen, Premarin, Estraderm, Oestradiol Implants and micronised Oestradiol (a component of Trisequens). There are, however, significant differences between the architecture of these various forms of oestrogen and the effects they have on the body. Some lower your blood pressure, while others do not alter it; some seem to affect moods more than others. These effects are especially pronounced in particular women.

When doctors talk of synthetic hormones, they are referring to hormones that are structurally different from those produced by the body and are not broken down or converted into other substances in the usual ways. One synthetic oestrogen widely prescribed for the treatment of menopausal symptoms until the mid-1980s, and still on the market, is Estigyn. This contains ethinyl oestradiol, a common component of the contraceptive pill and a far more powerful oestrogen, in terms of its effect on body tissues, than the natural oestrogens.

In recent years Estigyn has fallen from favour among specialist menopause clinicians because of increased stimulation of liver-derived proteins that may result in high blood pressure, fluid build-up, and an increase in clotting factors. In other words Estigyn, being synthetic, is capable of 'revving up' the liver far more than the natural oestrogens. A major reason why synthetic hormones are more likely to cause side effects than natural hormones is that the body takes longer to break them down, providing more time for them to act on various tissues. This effect may be enhanced with age, which is why doctors prefer not to use them in the older woman.

The natural oestrogens used in HRT formulations tend to have fewer effects on liver function (and consequently on blood pressure and blood clotting) than the synthetic oestrogens. They may be considered suitable if you are one of those women for whom the synthetic hormones of the Pill were not considered safe.

Women who are starting HRT for the first time some years after their menopause (whether it occurs naturally or as a result of medical treatment) should always be prescribed

✐ Dose reduction should be gradual when you are stopping HRT

natural forms of oestrogen, and the dose should be low initially and increased slowly if necessary. Start low and go slow is a wise motto for any hormone therapy. Examples of widely used natural and synthetic oestrogens, and the typical dosage range, are listed on page 175.

Lydia was sixty-two when she went onto HRT with a view to halting a worrying deterioration in bone density. This had been diagnosed by comparing the results of bone density scans performed when she was fifty-nine and then three years later. She was prescribed a dose of oestrogen usually given to women immediately after the menopause and developed sore breasts, excessive nipple sensitivity and nausea. Her doctor should have started her on a lower dose and slowly increased it over a period of three to six months. When Lydia was prescribed a natural oestrogen at a low dose, she experienced no worrying side effects, and for *her* this was a sufficient dose to stabilise bone density.

What are progesterone and progestogen?

During the fertile years progesterone is produced within the ovaries as a result of ovulation. It dampens down oestrogen's effect on the growth and thickening of the endometrium, the lining of the uterus. When the levels of oestrogen and progesterone decline towards the end of the menstrual cycle, the endometrium is shed as a menstrual bleed. The term progestogen is used to describe any manufactured substance that has similar chemical effects on the body to those of progesterone.

PROGESTOGENS USED IN HRT   Although all the progestogens used in HRT have properties similar to those of progesterone, the body breaks them down in rather different ways. They are all more powerful than progesterone too, having more pronounced effects when given at doses comparable to the levels of progesterone found in the body. (For a detailed description of the varieties of progestogen used in HRT see page 176.) The main reason for including progestogen in HRT is to protect the endometrium, the lining of the uterus. If the endometrium is exposed to constant oestrogen without progestogen, the endometrium may become too thick. This condition is known as hyperplasia, which occasionally develops into cancer.

It follows that, if you have had a hysterectomy, endometrial hyperplasia is not something for you to be concerned about. The way is clear for you to use an oestrogen-only form of HRT. This seems to be an option with few side effects or risks, but you must be carefully monitored.

Some women cannot tolerate the progestogen component of HRT as it can produce unwanted results such as breast tenderness, increased blood pressure, mood swings, depression, acne, backache, bloating and abdominal cramps. These symptoms resemble those of premenstrual syndrome. 'I hate progestogen,' said thirty-year-old Mardi, whose diseased ovaries were removed two years ago. She has since tried various combinations of oestrogen and progestogen, partly because of her mood changes. 'The progestogen makes me snappy and irrational and I get fed up with it. Some months I'm a bit naughty: I don't take the progestogen at all.'

At those times when Mardi has both progestogen and oestrogen she has regular withdrawal bleeds, that is, bleeding for a few days at a predictable time of the month. Withdrawal

> *More is known about HRT than ever before, but doctors are still on a learning curve with it*

bleeds are usually indistinguishable from short menstrual bleeds (they tend to be two to four days long) but, of course, they come about in different ways, being induced by hormone therapy. If you are taking progestogen you may also experience unpredictable bleeding, which is known as breakthrough bleeding. Understandably, such withdrawal bleeds and breakthrough bleeds deter some women from embarking on HRT or persevering with it, since an advantage of menopause for many women is an end to the bother of tampons and pads. A number of women appear to be happy to continue having

BEFORE DECIDING ON HRT . . .

You should have a thorough history and examination before beginning HRT. This should include all of the following:
- a full check of your general health, including the occurrence of any symptoms that may be related to menopause (hot flushes, headaches, vaginal dryness, for example), and an assessment of any social and psychological factors that may be contributing to your situation
- an assessment of your present and past menstrual cycle, including any changes to the pattern of your periods, their frequency, and the amount of blood loss
- a discussion of your lifestyle, including exercise and nutrition patterns and your use of medications, alcohol and cigarettes
- details of any previous medical, obstetrical, gynaecological or psychological symptoms, and any personal or family history of breast cancer or breast lumps, blood clot formation, heart attack or stroke, fractures or osteoporosis, uterine fibroids, endometriosis, problems experienced with the Pill, liver

withdrawal bleeds. The particular combination and timing of oestrogen and progestogen in HRT have a major influence on whether and when women experience bleeding. The bleeding patterns associated with various HRT formulations are discussed in more detail later in this chapter.

disease, any cessation of your menstrual periods for more than six months (unless caused by pregnancy and breastfeeding), and any experience of pre-menstrual symptoms
- weight and blood pressure measurements, an examination of the breasts and vagina (to check the cervix, uterus and ovaries), and a Pap smear if you have not had one within the past two years
- a mammogram, especially if you have a family or personal history of breast problems
- an assessment of blood fat levels (cholesterol and triglycerides) if this has not been made during the previous twelve months
- a bone density scan if, at any time during the fertile years, menstruation stopped unexpectedly for longer than six months; and also if you have used, or still use, steroids (for example, in asthma or thyroid treatment), have had a recent fracture, have a family history of fractures or osteoporosis, or for any reason regard bone density information as an important part of your decision about HRT

What is testosterone?

It is a hormone that contributes to feelings of wellbeing and to the maintenance of a woman's so-called 'secondary sexual characteristics' such as distribution of hair, type of voice, and libido. Although testosterone is usually thought of solely as a male sex hormone (also known as an androgen), this is incorrect. It is more accurately described as 'the third female sex hormone'. Women are already producing testosterone during childhood and continue to do so for the rest of their lives.

TESTOSTERONE AS PART OF HRT   If you have had your ovaries removed surgically, you may become aware of lethargy and loss of libido. The addition of testosterone to HRT, or perhaps testosterone on its own, may prove helpful in your case.

Diagnostic hysteroscopy

In some women, a procedure called a diagnostic hysteroscopy is in order when there is abnormal bleeding around the time of menopause, spontaneous bleeding after the menopause, or abnormal bleeding while on HRT. The purpose is to try to find the cause of the abnormal bleeding. The procedure involves the insertion of a small telescope through the cervix, which enables the doctor to view the endometrial tissue and assess its distribution and thickness and the presence of any abnormalities. At or after hysteroscopy the doctor can take a sample of the endometrium by means of biopsy or curettage. If you still have your uterus and are being prescribed, or choose to take, oestrogen without added progestogen (this is known as unopposed oestrogen), you should have an endometrial biopsy or a curette every six to twelve months. The same applies to women on HRT who have had previous abnormal changes to the endometrium.

Ways of administering HRT

Hormone therapy at menopause can come in the form of pills; skin patches; vaginal gels, tablets, pessaries or rings; implants; or injections.

PILLS In general, pills are the first-line hormone treatment for women at and after menopause. This form of HRT is usually cheaper than the alternatives, and the available research evidence about risks and benefits is more comprehensive for them. It also has the attraction of familiarity for women experienced with the Pill. A range of oestrogens and progestogens are available in tablet form (see pages 175–6). Reasons for choosing one rather than another will depend on your menopausal symptoms, your medical or family history, side effects experienced if and when you used the Pill, and your doctor's preference.

An increasing number of hormone varieties are produced in a micronised form that consists of tiny particles easily absorbed by the stomach and intestines. The constituents of the hormone pills then pass through the liver before reaching target tissues like the uterus, vagina and bones.

Advantages of the pill format include the ability to change the dosage or variety of hormone quickly, putting a rapid stop to side effects. This form of hormone therapy also tends to be less expensive than alternatives.

Disadvantages include the potential for gastro-intestinal problems such as nausea and the liver side effects discussed earlier. Those women still prescribed synthetic oestrogen may be at increased risk of high blood pressure and blood clot formation. Taking pills each day may also prove inconvenient if your life tends to be unpredictable and you are one of those people who find pill-taking hard to remember. It may help to put your pills in a place you can't overlook – in the tea caddy, for instance, if you always start the day with a cuppa, or next to the toothpaste.

SKIN PATCHES   Skin patches containing natural oestrogens are often prescribed to women who experience troublesome nausea and vomiting while taking oestrogen in pill form, or who are at risk of blood clot formation or high blood pressure from oral oestrogen therapy. In the US, where patches have been used for longer than in Australia, this is the method for about 40 per cent of women taking oestrogen after menopause.

They are transparent, come in a range of sizes depending on dosage (see page 176), and are applied to the abdomen, buttock or upper arm twice a week (for example, Monday morning and Thursday night).

Patches containing combinations of oestrogen and progestogen are also becoming available in an increasing number of countries, though not in Australia at the time of writing. The small and relatively constant doses of hormone released from patches and absorbed through the skin into the bloodstream more closely resemble the oestrogen and progesterone secretions of the body than do hormones taken in pill form.

Studies have confirmed their effectiveness in significantly reducing hot flushes, night sweats, vaginal dryness and urinary symptoms. Preliminary findings of other studies indicate that patches maintain bone density and reduce fracture rates, although long-term studies are needed to confirm this. There is also evidence that patches increase blood flow to the major blood vessels of the heart, but it is too early to say whether this translates to reduced rates of heart disease and heart attack.

Major **advantages** of the patches, compared with HRT pills, are their low rate of gastro-intestinal, bowel- and liver-related side effects, including blood pressure changes and blood clot abnormalities.

Disadvantages include skin reactions in some women, the cost (double that of pills), and the need to remember to change patches twice weekly. Skin irritation, which some studies indicate is a problem in up to 40 per cent of users, may be overcome by regularly changing the position of the patch on your body. Another thing to remember is that the site of

> *Using a patch allows the body to absorb oestrogen steadily and in small doses throughout the day and night, instead of all at once when a hormone pill is taken*

the patch may affect the rate of hormone absorption into your system. For example, if you place a patch on a part of your body that is moved frequently (such as the upper arm), your body will absorb it faster than if the patch is attached to your abdomen.

Sydney neurologists have described the case of a woman attending aerobics classes who experienced mysterious throbbing headaches, nausea and intermittent dizziness that were eventually traced to her hormone patches. Dr Kathryn North and Dr Llewelyn Davies, from the Royal Prince Alfred Hospital, said the headaches invariably started within an hour of her completing classes and did not improve when she switched from a 'high impact' to a 'low impact' exercise scheme. They feared initially that the woman, aged forty-eight, had a brain tumour. On further questioning her, the doctors realised that the onset of the post-exercise headaches coincided with a switch from oestrogen pills to patches. They suggested that the woman's aerobic activities were expanding the blood vessels under her skin, resulting in increased absorption of the hormone and the triggering of her headaches.

To test the theory, the woman removed the patch before each of her next six aerobic classes and the headaches ceased. When she exercised while wearing it, the headaches returned. 'Aerobics classes are popular in urban Australia', Drs North and Davies said in a letter to the international medical journal the *Lancet*. 'With the increasing use of transdermal oestrogen replacement therapy in postmenopausal women, this unusual headache may occur more often. Instruction from the prescriber will limit this disabling complication.'

There is a specified-purpose Pharmaceutical Benefits listing in Australia at approximately $15 a month for women who cannot tolerate oestrogen by mouth. Private prescriptions cost between $28 and $42 a month, depending on patch size.

VAGINAL CREAMS, TABLETS, PESSARIES AND RINGS

Oestrogen-containing vaginal preparations are often used by women in whom vaginal dryness makes sex distressingly painful. You may also benefit from these preparations if you have urinary symptoms such as a need to urinate frequently, or you experience recurrent urinary tract infections. Severe symptoms of this kind may need more far-reaching hormone therapy.

The oestrogen is absorbed into the bloodstream through the cells lining the vagina, and its major effect is in the immediate vicinity of the vagina and bladder. It is also carried to other parts of the body, including the uterus. For this reason, if you have an intact uterus and use vaginal creams, tablets or pessaries more than three times a week, you should probably be taking an oral progestogen for ten to fourteen days every three months. This ensures that any build-up of endometrial tissue is shed as a withdrawal bleed or, if no bleeding occurs, it provides reassurance that the endometrium is not in any danger.

Hormone rings, which sit in the top of the vagina for three months before needing to be replaced, release a small and constant stream of oestrogen that is absorbed by the cells of the vagina and cervix. Once again, if your uterus is intact you should take a ten-to-fourteen-day course of progestogen

> *'One size fits all' is not an appropriate way to approach HRT. Women's needs are as varied as women themselves*

every three months to ensure that stimulation of the endometrium does not occur. These devices are on trial in Australia at the time of writing.

Advantages of these forms of local therapy include a concentrated dose of oestrogen at the site of the symptom rather than its widespread dispersal through the body.

Disadvantages include the lack of effect on other menopausal symptoms (such as hot flushes and night sweats); the rare occurrence of unexpected spotting or bleeding or endometrial hyperplasia (excessive thickening of the uterine lining) if used too frequently without added progestogen; their messiness; and the embarrassment felt by some women about putting things into their vaginas.

IMPLANTS   Another HRT option (oestrogen with or without testosterone – which may be suggested for boosting your libido) is insertion under the skin of pellets containing one or more hormones. The pellet is usually placed in the fat of the lower abdomen, buttock or upper thigh, and a replacement is inserted every three to twelve months, depending on the dose required. This small and simple surgical procedure is performed in the doctor's rooms or at a menopause clinic.

The amount of hormone absorbed from the implant varies according to how long it has been there, its position (for example, more hormone is absorbed if the implant is in the upper arm of a swimmer than if it is placed in a buttock), its depth under the skin (the deeper the implant, the greater the absorption), physical activity levels (exercise increases blood flow) and the presence of inflammation or scar tissue around the implant.

Women who find implants useful include those who for one reason or another cannot tolerate oestrogen in pill or patch form, and those needing large doses of oestrogen. These advantages may offset a common problem with implants, which is that the dose of hormone entering the body is initially high and reduces with time.

For example Natalie, a young woman who had an artificial menopause following cancer treatment, required relatively

> *Implants continue releasing oestrogen well after their 'use by' date. If you have a uterus, you should still be on progestogen for one to three years after the last insertion*

large amounts of oestrogen to alleviate recurring bouts of severe hot flushes. She found the implant both more convenient and more effective than pills, although she experienced sore breasts for some weeks after the implant was inserted (a higher than average hormone dose was entering her body), and a return of flushes as the time for a replacement implant approached (the hormone dose released by the implant had dropped significantly).

Many doctors believe that oestrogen implants should not be used as first-line HRT in women who have a uterus. This is because implants deliver substantially higher levels of oestrogen than other HRT formulations (at least part of the time) and, while helping women to feel wonderful, these levels can greatly increase the risk of severe, uncontrollable bleeding and possible hysterectomy. According to Dr John Eden from the University of New South Wales, some women on oestrogen implants feel a euphoria similar to that experienced by men on anabolic steroids. 'But women pay a price if they have a uterus; they run the risk of heavy, uncontrollable periods.' In the case of Margo, a patient with fibroids who had an implant inserted, the bleeding was so heavy that hysterectomy was the only option. 'You rarely see this with other therapies, because the oestrogen levels are relatively low', Dr Eden says. 'Women with fibroids may get irregular bleeds, but you don't see the activation and growth that you may get with an implant.'

It is extremely important that any woman with an intact uterus who is using an oestrogen implant realises the necessity of teaming progestogen with it for one to three years *after* the last implant is inserted. Implants continue to release small amounts of oestrogen for a very long time after their 'use by' date. It is unwise to discontinue the progestogen until two to three months after withdrawal bleeds have stopped.

An **advantage** of implants is their convenience, with no need to remember a daily pill or twice-weekly patch.

In most cases GPs are the best advisers on the menopause and HRT

Disadvantages include the occasional rejection by the body of an implant, indicated by scar tissue formation around it and perhaps its eventual expulsion; and the necessity for a small surgical procedure each time an implant is inserted or taken out. This may create problems in remote areas if the implant has to be removed quickly, either because of intolerable side effects or the diagnosis of a serious medical condition likely to be aggravated by hormone therapy. A possible disadvantage is the upfront cost of the implant and its insertion. Over time, however, it may be no more costly than patches or pills.

A small number of women with oestradiol implants experience an earlier than normal return of their symptoms – as if the implant had run out – despite adequate levels of oestrogen in their blood. These women return for further implants at shorter and shorter intervals. The cause of this phenomenon, called tachyphylaxis, is not known. With each implant inserted, the amount of oestradiol in the blood rises, usually to high levels. Though the consequences of persistently high levels are unknown, further implants are not recommended until levels return to the normal premenopausal range. Affected women go through a difficult withdrawal phase and require regular blood tests until normal levels are attained. If their symptoms are severe, relief may be obtained with the higher-dose oestrogen patches. Regular testing of oestradiol levels will help to avoid this phenomenon in implant users.

INJECTIONS As discussed earlier in this chapter, testosterone sometimes forms part of HRT. Some doctors prefer to administer testosterone therapy by injection rather than by implant because the dosage can more easily be adjusted to meet your individual needs. Injections of oestrogen and progestogen may also prove helpful in controlling symptoms of menopause, especially if you are a woman who cannot tolerate pill forms of oestrogen or progestogen.

Hormone combinations and single-drug formats

Books about menopause often seem to imply that the only forms of HRT available are Premarin (an oestrogen isolated from the urine of pregnant mares) and Provera (a progestogen of long standing). It is certainly true that the most common mix of hormones prescribed as HRT is an oestrogen (taken in every day by pill, patch or implant), plus a progestogen (taken daily for ten to fourteen days, then not used for the rest of the month), but the numerous options available mean that hormone formats can be tailored to meet each woman's needs.

COMBINED CYCLICAL THERAPY Many varieties of oestrogen and progestogen (see pages 175–6) can be used in this combined hormone format, referred to as cyclical progestogen. The oestrogen component is the main agent for relieving menopausal symptoms, while the addition of a certain amount of progestogen puts the brakes on growth of the endometrium. A withdrawal bleed occurs when you stop taking progestogen.

There is variability in the types of oestrogen and progestogen prescribed, and these hormones may be taken together in a single pill or patch, or separately. For women taking separate hormone pills (for example, because the doctor wants to use dosages not found in the available combined-pill formats), an easy way to remember when to start the progestogen is at the beginning of each calendar month. The progestogen is then stopped on the tenth, twelfth or fourteenth day of the month (depending on the doctor's instructions). You could, on the other hand, use a 'calendar dial pack', which contains ten oestrogen-plus-progestogen tablets followed by eighteen oestrogen pills.

You can expect a withdrawal bleed to begin anywhere

between the tenth day of taking progestogen and a week after it is finished. If bleeding starts outside this time (that is, before day ten or after day seventeen, nineteen or twenty-one, depending on how many days the progestogen is taken), it is likely that the hormone dose is inadequate and needs to be altered. Most women taking progestogen for ten to fourteen days a month (that is, cyclical progestogen) have a withdrawal bleed each month at the end of the progestogen phase. The first few bleeds tend to be heavier than later bleeds. In about 50 per cent of women taking this cyclical progestogen, withdrawal bleeds disappear after about ten years; in most other users, withdrawal bleeds continue for however long the hormones are taken, usually becoming lighter with time.

In a small proportion of users, of whom Marita is an example, cyclical progestogen therapy never causes bleeding. The absence of bleeding after she started taking oestrogen and progestogen caused Marita some initial concern, but she was reassured by her doctor that nothing was amiss. She then wondered whether she needed to take progestogen at all, but her doctor impressed on her the necessity of continuing with this part of the therapy as she still had a uterus, which would be at increased risk of abnormal tissue growth, and possibly cancer, if she took oestrogen alone. Provera is the progestogen best documented as preventing abnormal growth of the endometrium.

CONTINUOUS COMBINED HRT   A second common oestrogen–progestogen combination involves taking both hormones every day. This is described as continuous combined HRT. Individual doses of progestogen are lower than when the progestogen is taken for ten to fourteen days a month, but the total monthly intake is similar. If progestogen gives you side effects like those of premenstrual syndrome (such as irritability and breast tenderness) you may find this hormone format helpful. About 80 to 90 per cent of users of this continuous combined HRT no longer experience withdrawal bleeds after an interval of six to twelve months. However, irregular bleeding may occur for the first few months, and women with fibroids may have irregular bleeding that is difficult to control without surgery. There is some research to suggest that continuous combined HRT may have a less stimulatory effect on breast cells and breast cancer than combined cyclical therapy or oestrogen alone. This is a matter of continuing controversy that is discussed in further detail in chapter 4.

Freda, whose principal reason for being on HRT was control of severe hot flushes, was pleased with the effect on her bleeding patterns of swapping from one HRT routine to another. Her experience of cyclical progestogen therapy was unacceptable. 'I was still having moderate to heavy with-

Once you find a format and dosage of hormones that suits you, there is generally no need to change

drawal bleeds sixteen months after I started and I felt these were more of a nuisance than the hot flushes. My doctor then suggested I try continuous combined HRT and, after three months of intermittent spotting and seven months of withdrawal bleeds, I no longer had any bleeding and felt well.'

As with combined cyclical therapy, women on continuous combined HRT who do not have withdrawal bleeds are considered to be at no higher risk of endometrial cancer than women who bleed, and should continue with progestogen as recommended by their doctor.

OESTROGEN ALONE   With one exception, oestrogen on its own in any form is considered safe only if you no longer have a uterus. Since about 30 per cent of Australian women have had a hysterectomy by the age of sixty-five, the number of potential users of this relatively straightforward form of HRT is large. The exception is women with an intact uterus whose menopausal problems are confined to vaginal dryness, urinary frequency or recurring urinary tract infections. If this is your situation, you can use oestrogen alone in the form of vaginal creams, tablets or pessaries two or three times a week (*but no more frequently*) after using it for seven to ten days in a row initially if your doctor so advises. If vaginal or urinary symptoms are still quite troublesome, this form of therapy may be inadequate and you may be advised to consider a hormone format (for example oestrogen pills) that will have more widespread effects on the body.

It is very important, if you have an intact uterus and are using oestrogen creams, tablets or pessaries intermittently in your vagina without added progestogen for an extended time, to be assessed by a doctor at least every six to twelve months. Monitoring is necessary because endometrial hyperplasia

> *Women who no longer have a uterus are the easiest to treat with HRT because oestrogen on its own is all that is required*

(excessive thickening of the uterine lining) and subsequent endometrial cancer may occur after some years if the oestrogen dose is too high. Even a single spot of vaginal blood could indicate a problem and should immediately trigger a visit to your doctor.

HIGH-DOSE PROGESTOGEN ALONE For reasons that are unclear, high doses of progestogen alone may prove helpful in relieving the problem of hot flushes if you are one of those women for whom oestrogen has not been recommended (such as those with a personal experience of breast cancer).

TESTOSTERONE ALONE OR COMBINED WITH OESTROGEN AND PROGESTOGEN Testosterone alone or combined with other hormones may be given to women concerned about their loss of libido when this does not seem to be caused by psychosocial factors or discord with a partner. Testosterone is usually given by implant six-monthly or by injection into muscle tissue every three to six weeks. The dosage by implant is about one-quarter that prescribed for men with libido problems.

What stage are you at?

If you are having irregular, heavy and prolonged menstrual periods and distressing menopausal symptoms
Your hormone therapy options include the following:
- HRT pill that combines oestrogen and progestogen
- natural oestrogen daily plus progestogen for ten to fourteen days a month
- low-dose combined Pill for women needing contraception
- the synthetic oestrogen ethinyl oestradiol, in combination with the progestogen-like substance cyproterone acetate (the combined formulation Diane-35) if acne and worrisome hair growth are problems and contraception is also needed

If you are postmenopausal and have a uterus
Your options for hormone therapy include the following:
- natural oestrogen pill daily or continous oestrogen by patch

or implant, teamed with progestogen for ten to fourteen days a month (combined cyclical therapy)
- continuous natural oestrogen and continuous progestogen (continuous combined HRT)

The first of these approaches usually causes monthly withdrawal bleeds that become lighter after a few months and may continue for however long you use HRT. With the second approach, irregular bleeding may occur for the first few months but most women no longer have any bleeding a year later.

If you are postmenopausal and do not have a uterus
Your options for hormone therapy include the following:
- natural oestrogen by pill daily or continuous oestrogen by patch or implant
- natural oestrogen daily and low-dose progestogen daily (for about six months immediately after surgery for endometriosis)
- oestrogen with or without testosterone implants

Dosages

The HRT dosage prescribed depends on a number of factors such as its purpose (for example, mainly for symptom control or mainly for reducing the risk of later heart or fracture problems) and a woman's individual response to it. The oestrogen dosages needed to relieve symptoms may be higher or lower than those required to provide long-term protection against heart disease and osteoporosis, depending on the severity of symptoms. Women on HRT before menopause is confirmed cannot rely on it for contraception as hormone dosages are insufficient to prevent pregnancy. As explained previously, a low-dose combined Pill is one way of obtaining both the benefits of HRT and contraceptive protection.

Whether it is taken every day or for ten to fourteen days per cycle, the total monthly dose of progestogen in HRT is similar to that given to a woman on the Pill. The dosage used by Tessa, who is taking progestogen daily, was arrived at by lowering the daily dose until she had breakthrough bleeding, then adjusting upwards.

Individual variability in the body's capacity to deal with the hormones of HRT is another reason why a dose that relieves symptoms in one woman has little effect on another. In the case of hormone patches and implants, the position on or in the body affects the amount of hormone the body absorbs and therefore the dosage required.

When a doctor is deciding on the most suitable dosage or hormone format for you, your individual response will be crucial. The hormones used initially may not relieve your symptoms adequately, or they may have unwanted effects. It may then be necessary to change the kind of oestrogen or progestogen used, or to alter the dose.

Timing

There is some evidence to suggest that when progestogen is given for ten to fourteen days per cycle to women prior to menopause, it should be taken in phase with the existing menstrual cycle if it is still apparent. This helps to reduce the occurrence of breakthrough bleeding. The experience of Josie, who developed severe hot flushes at the age of forty-five while still menstruating regularly, illustrates the point. Her cycle length had always fluctuated around twenty-one days, and when she took progestogen for the first twelve days of each month she experienced repeated breakthrough bleeding that required investigation.

At first her doctor tried manipulating the dose and type of oestrogen and progestogen, but this did not help. Finally, her doctor twigged to the possibility that the bleeding problems could be due to the fact that the hormones her ovaries were still producing intermittently were not synchronising with the

> *If you use HRT before menopause is confirmed, you cannot rely on it for contraception. You will need to use another form of contraception in the meantime*

hormones she was taking on HRT. Josie was advised to take the last progestogen tablet on the day before the start of the next menstrual bleed she was expecting. Thus, with a twenty-one-day menstrual cycle, she took the progestogen from day nine to day twenty. This simple alteration resulted in much less breakthrough bleeding.

The regular medical check-up

It usually takes six months for side effects associated with HRT to settle. A doctor will normally start with an 'off-the-shelf' hormone format and then make adjustments to suit your particular responses. Two months after starting on HRT you should be reviewed by your doctor, with a follow-up three months later. Once-yearly checks are appropriate from then on, unless side effects or other concerns like irregular bleeding occur, in which case prompt investigation is in order. Also make sure you ask your doctor to check your breasts and to confirm that you are not overdue for a mammogram.

Once a format and dosage of hormones that suit your individual needs are found, it is usual to stay with this formula for as long as HRT is required.

Duration of HRT

The length of time for a woman to have HRT remains a matter of debate. Most doctors advise patients to continue the therapy until a break from their hormone format no longer results in troublesome symptoms. This generally occurs in one to three years, but sometimes five, ten or even fifteen years.

If HRT is given solely to reduce a perceived risk of osteoporosis or heart disease, current evidence suggests that the longer the use, the greater the benefit. It seems that at least five years of HRT are needed to obtain a statistically significant benefit for the bones or heart, and to get maximum benefit you need from fifteen years to lifetime therapy. Bone density measurements (see chapter 3) may give helpful information when the question arises of whether or not to continue with HRT. If the bone density is excellent and menopausal symptoms are no longer troubling, you may wish to stop HRT pending a review of your situation (including another bone density measurement) in two to three years time. If the bone density is of concern and there are no compelling reasons to discontinue HRT, staying on the therapy is the best course.

If the main consideration prompting HRT was abnormal blood fat levels, an improvement to normal in cholesterol and triglyceride levels does not provide a convincing reason for stopping it. Indeed, it may be an argument for persisting with the therapy as it is doing the job required.

CHAPTER 3

The benefits

WOMEN CONSIDER HRT for many different reasons, the most common being to relieve symptoms associated with the menopause. In addition, women at risk of fractures due to osteoporosis, or likely to develop heart and blood vessel disease, may have HRT recommended to them by their medical practitioners. The same advice is increasingly given to women with existing osteoporosis, or those with a diagnosed heart or blood vessel condition, the rationale being that HRT may prevent these problems getting any worse.

HRT and menopausal symptom control

Hot flushes and sweating often prompt menopausal women to seek medical assistance. Other common reasons for consultations include psychological symptoms like loss of concentration and 'feeling blue', general tiredness, irritability, vaginal dryness and pain with intercourse, loss of libido, urinary frequency and persistent urinary discomfort.

FLUSHES AND SWEATS Approximately 40 per cent of women in the Melbourne Women's Midlife Health Study who had a natural menopause between the ages of forty-five and fifty-five experienced hot flushes and night sweats around this time. This figure, lower than reported in many other studies, reinforces the need to study non-clinic populations of women as well as those with a greater burden of symptoms, many of whom have had a premature menopause with or without medical intervention.

In the early menopause group, the incidence of hot flushes may reach 70 per cent or more. Insomnia, which affected about 40 per cent of menopausal women in the Melbourne study, is sometimes due to a woman waking repeatedly in the night, drenched from heavy sweating. The distressing combination of night sweats and insomnia may interfere with sexual interest and activity as well as making it more difficult to cope with the following day and its pressures.

Pauline was prescribed tranquillisers by the first doctor she consulted about her problems of night sweats and insomnia. 'I told the doctor how I'd wake in the early hours of the morning in a lather, I'd toss and turn and still not get back to sleep. In the process I'd disturb my husband, who'd get cranky because he had a lot on his plate at the time. He'd growl at me and snarl during breakfast.' Pauline finally consulted another doctor, who reassured her that the night sweats would probably become less intense and disappear over a few years. She explained the situation to her husband and discussed ways of minimising the night-time disturbance – including fewer bedclothes, more fresh air in the bedroom, and a spare nightgown in the bathroom, just in case.

Women know that the menopause brings flushes and sweats, and generally cope if they are not too frequent. For some women, however, they happen so often and are so severe that they tend to dominate life. Amandine Dupin (better known as the French novelist George Sand) was forty-nine when she wrote in a private letter, dated 1853, 'I am as well as I can be, given the crisis of my age. So far everything has taken place without grave consequence, but with sweats that I find overwhelming, and which are laughable because they are imaginary. I experience the phenomenon of believing that I am sweating fifteen or twenty times a day and night . . . I have both the heat and the fatigue. I wipe my face with a white handkerchief and it is laughable because I am not sweating at all. However, that makes me very tired.'

As many women can testify, hot flushes and sweating episodes are far from imaginary, being intimately associated with fluxing levels in certain hormones and a rise in skin temperature by several degrees. Some women have accompanying nausea and palpitations. Flushes tend to be more prevalent in women who experience a rapid change in sex hormone levels, for example following a hysterectomy and bilateral salpingo-oophorectomy (that is, removal of both ovaries as well as the uterus and cervix), than in women who have a natural menopause. Flushes and sweats are also more likely in women who smoke, have a history of premenstrual syndrome (commonly abbreviated to PMS) or experience flushes and night sweats before menopause.

The duration of these problems may also influence a woman's decision to seek medical help. Flushes and sweats that disappear after a few months are easier to cope with than the same symptoms lasting for years. Studies show that flushes go on for about two years in most of the women affected. About 20 per cent have them for five or more years, and about 10 per cent are still having occasional flushes into their sixties. Descriptions of flushing and sweating episodes vary enormously. Some women tell us that their hot flushes are like a spray of hot oil that quickly passes. Others note that the sensation of heat is inevitably followed by shivering and cold sweats. Yet other descriptions of night sweats make them sound like clammy journeys through tropical rainforests without the beautiful surroundings, the aftermath of which is a need to change sheets and nightwear.

A combination of oestrogen and progestogen may be recommended for dealing with hot flushes and night sweats if

After starting HRT many women find that their concentration improves, confidence returns, decision-making seems easier, and they regain their old zip

you still have your uterus. When the uterus has been removed, the use of oestrogen alone is considered a safe way to reduce the impact of flushes. High doses of progestogen alone are occasionally helpful in controlling them, but this approach is usually suggested only if oestrogen therapy is not recommended or tolerated.

Any doctor who prescribes HRT to help women with flushes will know that this symptom responds very well to oestrogen, often within a week. If you are a woman with debilitating or embarrassing flushes, the possibility of getting relief in such a short time may be persuasive. Some questions remain, however, about how much of the benefit is due to HRT and how much to the psychological support the doctor provides.

Research shows that a significant number of women experience improvements in flush frequency and severity when they take a medication lacking any active ingredient. This is known as a placebo response — that is, the patient's symptoms are relieved when a harmless substance, like a sugar pill, is substituted for a biologically active agent. Too few studies of menopausal therapies, of both the prescribed and 'alternative' kind, have been sufficiently well designed to separate the effectiveness of the therapy from a woman's response to the empathy, support and interest shown by her practitioner. Of three major studies of oestrogen therapy for hot flushes that have taken the placebo response into account, all have demonstrated an improvement.

PSYCHOLOGICAL SYMPTOMS In surveys of women seeking medical help at and around menopause, about one woman in four reports psychological symptoms including poor concentration, faulty memory, loss of confidence, uncharacteristic sadness and difficulty making decisions. There has been speculation that lowered oestrogen levels are the cause of such symptoms by a direct effect on the output of chemicals involved in message transmission in the brain (called neurotransmitters). It is difficult to separate the effects of hormones from other factors that may influence psychological symptoms, such as stress at home or work, lifestyle modifications to do with diet and exercise, and major life changes.

Supporting the impression that this disquiet among women is not simply a matter of hormone levels, the Melbourne Women's Midlife Health Study found no apparent association between mental wellbeing and whether women were still having regular periods or had reached menopause. The differences in the findings of various studies may relate to the groups being studied: women who attend medical practitioners for help may well be more psychologically stressed than random samples of middle-aged women. In the Melbourne study, involving 2000 randomly selected women aged forty-five to fifty-five, those who felt mentally well were more likely to have low levels of stress in their lives, a positive attitude to ageing and to menopause, to exercise vigorously, to live with a partner, to be in good general health and to be a non-smoker. Women should first consider whatever non-medical steps they can take to reduce day-to-day stress. A daily walk, a regular game of tennis or an aerobics class might do the trick.

The relationship between psychological symptoms and the menopause is evidently far from straightforward. A complex interplay of factors affects psychological functioning – among them personality, hormone changes, alterations in social and family stresses, the presence or absence of physical illnesses, and perhaps also feelings of loss and grief at entering the final third of life and realising the inevitability of death. To make

> *The interaction between ageing, the menopause and mood changes is complex. The extent to which physical and psychological symptoms are directly related to altered hormone levels remains speculative*

the situation even less clear, there will always be a small group of women with severe psychiatric illnesses, who just happen to be menopausal at the time their illness comes to prominence.

Additionally, psychological symptoms blamed on menopause are inclined to show placebo responses: as we explained earlier, the symptoms may be relieved almost as well by a dud pill as by a prescribed product, arguably because part of the 'healing therapy' is the extra support and interest the patient is receiving.

The medical literature is probably best summarised by stating that whereas there is little evidence for an association between menopause and fully developed psychiatric disease, such as clinical depression, less severe psychological upsets seem to affect some women as they approach menopause or soon afterwards. HRT seems to relieve this state of affairs and to heighten a woman's sense of wellbeing. Thus many women on HRT experience improvements in their psychological functioning (concentration improves, confidence is restored, decision-making seems easier) and regain a spring in their step.

MOOD CHANGES   Many women feel they are changing personality during menopause, like the female equivalent of Dr Jekyll and Mr Hyde. Germaine Greer likens it to 'the person you know being stuffed inside a new one. The most unnerving, even terrifying, change is a sudden horrible propensity to blind rage . . . She finds herself calling down horrible vengeance and uttering mad threats, which seem to be throttled out of her, as if she was being squeezed in a giant hand. Sometimes the outburst is accompanied by a feeling of physical anxiety, amounting to pain, or a feeling of unbearable pressure in the head, or behind the eyes.' The choking rage is usually followed by 'exhaustion, helpless guilt and a futile wishing that whatever it was had not happened'.

The hormone replacement advocate Dr Robert A. Wilson (see chapter 2) linked the mood changes in his 'gentle, almost angelic mother' to his later efforts to find a 'treatment' for menopause. 'At the time I could not understand it. What was a boy in his teens to make of a phrase like "change of life"? . . . Yet something terrible was obviously happening. I was appalled at the transformation of the vital, wonderful woman who had been the dynamic focal point of our family into a pain-wracked, petulant individual. I could feel the deep wounds her senseless rages inflicted on my father, myself and the younger children. It was this frightful experience that later directed my interest as a physician to the problem of the menopause.'

Little is understood about why these mood swings occur, seemingly without conscious intent or reflection. One theory proposes a direct role for the fluxing ovarian hormones, the brain being one of the organs influenced by oestrogen. Others link menopausal mood swings with the relationship stresses that often occur during this life stage; the expectations, attitudes and personality of the woman; and influences like culture, social class and employment. Then again, maybe there is a biological explanation for mood swings.

Germaine Greer suggests that menopause may put 'women back in touch with their anger after thirty-five years of censorship by oestrogen'. She adds that the middle-aged female employer (one could add executive, wife or mother), dealing with people who ignore what she says on the basis that she is menopausal, is quite likely to have to think of a number of strategies to get their attention. 'A good deal of the anxiety of the middle-aged woman is caused by her awareness that she is turning into some kind of a harridan, a scold, a fishwife, but if you can't get attention any other way, what are you to do?'

Other unproven hypotheses for mood changes have shifted the focus to environmental factors. These include allergies to foods and petrochemical products, and the accumulation in bones during adolescence and early adulthood of lead, which is then released into tissues and blood with the onset of menopausal bone loss.

Studies of the effects of hormone therapy on personality suggest that use of oestrogen may moderate mood swings and cause women to become more agreeable. A recent Oxford University study found that oestrogen in the form of implants reduced shifts in mood, possibly because of changes in neurotransmitter function in the brain.

SKIN, MUSCLE AND JOINTS   There is evidence that low oestrogen levels over a period of years affect the collagen component of skin, causing it to become thinner, drier, more prone to damage, bruising and itching, and somewhat transparent in appearance. Loss of collagen also occurs in ligaments and other soft tissues, and this may explain joint aches and pains. An estimated 15 to 30 per cent of collagen is lost from the skin within five years of menopause. Another problem experienced by some women around this time is a crawling sensation on the skin (known as formication).

HRT appears to prevent the thinning effect or, if it has already occurred, to restore skin thickness and improve its texture by increasing the collagen content. It may also provide relief from crawling skin sensations, and muscle and joint aches and pains. All the hormone therapy in the world will not remove wrinkles, but they may become less noticeable while you are on HRT because the skin looks fuller. Hair texture may also improve, although there is not necessarily an increase in the number of hairs.

PALPITATIONS AND HEADACHES   You may be one of the many women who experience palpitations and headaches around the time of menopause. A Dutch study found that one in four women had palpitations at menopause, and headaches affect nearly a third of Australian-born women aged forty-five to fifty-five. For reasons that are not clear, some women have more frequent and severe tension-type headaches around menopause; for others, headaches, and particularly migraine, become less of a problem. Oestrogen appears to be effective in treating palpitations. It may alleviate migraine in some postmenopausal women too.

ENERGY LEVELS.   Women at midlife sometimes claim

that their get up and go has got up and gone. They can't raise the energy to pursue activities they have enjoyed for years. Such a woman is Bronwyn, whose youthfulness comes from an appetite for adventure that was unquenchable until menopause hit. 'I don't have flushes and I generally feel OK, except that I don't have any energy. I'm working near to home but I find it harder than ever to get up in the morning, and to get moving. The worst thing is that I just want to rest on my days off, instead of visiting friends or taking off for the bush. I haven't been able to look my hiking boots in the eye.'

If this is your scenario too, it is important – before allowing a doctor to reach for the prescription pad – to establish that your loss of energy has a physical origin and is not explained by job frustration or dissatisfaction, or the need for new challenges in life. Once you are satisfied that there is a physical basis to the problem, it is essential to have a check on your general health, diet, activity levels and lifestyle stresses before even considering HRT. Some women do find that energy levels respond to HRT. It is unclear to what extent this is due to an effect of HRT in settling other symptoms such as night sweats and sleeplessness; a feeling of wellbeing induced by HRT's action on the brain and other body tissues; or a placebo effect activated by a doctor's interest in and support of his or her patient.

SEX LIFE   Like psychological problems, sexual difficulties around the menopausal years are complex because they are affected by a wide range of social, environmental and interpersonal influences that may have little or nothing to do with menopause. The Melbourne Women's Midlife Health Study found that sexual interest and activity did not change significantly in about 62 per cent of women who had had a natural menopause, while 31 per cent reported that they felt less sexually interested, had sex less often, and found it more painful than previously. Approximately 7 per cent said they were more sexually interested and active, and some attributed this to a new partner in their lives.

Since sexual activities involve two partners, it is important not to assume that difficulties originate on the female side. As men age they tend to experience increasing problems with libido, erections, orgasmic capacity and penile sensitivity. This may compromise their sexual interest or capabilities. When Leah was fifty-seven, her husband Brian, aged sixty-four, suffered a heart attack. Although he was soon back at work, his sex drive all but disappeared and he had difficulty getting an erection. During counselling sessions he revealed that he feared dying during sexual activity, and that this weighed heavily on his mind.

In other couples, sex literally becomes a bruising experience. Some, but not all, women experience vaginal dryness and thinning of the vaginal lining after menopause, and this may make intercourse painful. This symptom is more frequent among postmenopausal women than their younger sisters, but is not confined to the postmenopause. A study of women in the south-east of England found that 40 per cent had this problem after menopause, but 26 per cent of premenopausal women also did. If the problem of painful intercourse becomes established, it can lead to lack of confidence in both partners and things may go from bad to worse.

This chapter looks specifically at the role of HRT, but hormone therapy is certainly not the whole answer to sexual difficulties around the time of menopause. There is some evidence that sexual problems will respond to HRT by its direct effect on vaginal lubrication, the vaginal lining (causing it to resume its former thickness), blood vessels and blood flow in the vagina, vulva and uterus, and perhaps also transmission of messages along nerve pathways to the genital organs. Oestrogen and testosterone seem to be the only hormone therapies that improve libido in women, although they are not universally effective.

Before embarking on HRT in the hope that it will improve your sex life, it is important that you explain the problem to your doctor in detail. Specialised sex therapy may be required, no matter how good your response to hormones, since the problem may have set in train patterns of sexual behaviour that are difficult to undo. You will find HRT and your sex life discussed in more detail in chapter 5.

LOWER URINARY TRACT PROBLEMS   Urinary frequency (going to the toilet more often), the pressing urge to go (known as urgency), and bladder incontinence (escape of urine when the need to urinate is very strong or when coughing or sneezing occurs) are more likely with increasing age and may be accentuated at menopause. Studies indicate that up to 50 per cent of women attending menopause clinics have some lower urinary tract symptoms. Treatment with HRT may relieve some of these symptoms, including urinary incontinence, frequency and urgency, by increasing the collagen of the urethra and vagina, and by improving muscle tone in the pelvic floor.

HRT and osteoporosis

Osteoporosis, a serious medical condition characterised by bones that are weak and tend to fracture, affects a third to a half of Australian women during their lifetime. (It is sometimes confused with osteoarthritis, but these are two completely different conditions.) There is conflicting information about when bone loss starts, but most of the evidence suggests that much of the damage occurs during and immediately after menopause. This loss of bone makes fractures more likely, but it takes a while to cause problems. Most women who experience a fracture don't have it until after the age of seventy, although about one in five do so earlier. Overall, between a third and a half of women have a fracture eventually, with spinal vertebrae, hips and wrists being most likely to be damaged.

The pain of a fracture can be severe and, to add insult to injury, vertebral fractures can reduce height. Marion suffered a series of spontaneous vertebral fractures in her seventies that reduced her height from 170 cm to 160 cm in a matter of years. Despite doing everything possible to stand erect, even using a back brace much of the time, she also developed a hump on the spine below her neck (sometimes called a dowager's hump).

Hip fractures tend to be even more debilitating, with a significant number of women who suffer this injury never leaving hospital. Recovery may involve surgery and extensive rehabilitation. The inability to return home, heart-breaking for many, may reflect the lack of quality, affordable home care services suitable for elderly women on the road to recovery but wishing to live alone, as well as the difficulties involved in gaining mobility after hip repair surgery.

The most marked rate of bone loss – up to 15 per cent in total – occurs in the first five to six years after menopause, followed by a slower decline. If you have an early menopause (natural or surgical), your risk of osteoporosis will increase: the earlier the menopause, the longer the time available for osteoporosis to develop.

Whether bones ever reach the stage of being fracture-prone depends on many factors, including your age (and thus how long bone loss has been occurring), how strong your bones were to start with (that is, your peak bone mass, which is usually achieved between the ages of twenty and thirty), and the rate of bone loss (this varies considerably among healthy women). Two bone density measurements taken a year apart will provide you with a good indication of whether or not you are at risk of osteoporosis.

The rapid loss of bone density typical of the first few years after menopause seems to be related to an increased rate of calcium and collagen loss from bones, probably due to oestrogen lack, and a reduced ability of the body to absorb calcium from food. But many other factors appear to be involved. No one knows why the sudden loss of bone density occurs soon after menopause, or why the rate of bone loss

> *Oestrogen in the form of pills, patches or implants, and oestrogen combined with a progestogen, seem to benefit bone health. The longer women are on hormone therapy, the stronger their bones*

reaches a plateau within a few years. Another finding that researchers are puzzling over is the rapid loss of bone in some women and the much slower loss in others. Whatever the reasons for such differences, HRT at menopause significantly lessens the loss of calcium from bones so that they remain strong for longer. Most efforts to investigate hormone therapy and osteoporosis have used oestrogen alone in pill form and in doses higher than are used today. Recent research indicates that progestogen also directly stimulates growth and development of bone-forming cells.

The link between osteoporosis and oestrogen levels was first recognised in 1941. Some years later, the effect of ovary removal on increased osteoporosis risk was observed and the beneficial effects of oestrogens on bone preservation confirmed.

The central role of oestrogen levels on osteoporosis and the success of oestrogen therapy in preventing menopausal bone loss and in reducing fracture risk is now widely accepted. Also recognised is the importance of an adequate dose of oestrogen if bone loss is to be prevented. Treatment with oestrogen remains the only form of therapy proven to reduce fracture rates in both the spine and hip. Some uncertainties remain about the way that oestrogen maintains bone strength.

The development of safe, acceptable and accurate techniques that measure bone mass at sites such as the spine and hip has contributed a great deal to the diagnosis and management of osteoporosis.

The methods used to assess the strength of bones provide information about their mineral content or their density, and the two are closely linked. These methods include single and dual photon absorptiometry, quantitative CT scan, heel bone ultrasound, and dual energy x-ray absorptiometry (often abbreviated to DEXA), words that are gobbledegook to just about everyone except the technicians who service the instruments involved.

If your bone strength is determined by single photon absorptiometry, you will be asked to immerse your forearm in a water bath and grasp a circular rod for about ten minutes, while a gamma ray source and detector scan your wrist bones. If dual photon absorptiometry is chosen, you will have to lie on a couch for about twenty minutes while a mechanical arm scans from above. In recent years DEXA has become the preferred method for measuring bone strength in the spine and hip because of its low radiation dose and speed of measurement.

At the time of writing the cost of the DEXA procedure varied from about $65 to $140. Some doctors advocate the use of bone density measurements at regular intervals for women with low bone densities in order to assess the response to HRT and to encourage them to remain on it.

FACTORS CONTRIBUTING TO OSTEOPOROSIS Recent UK research suggests that, although our health is generally better than that of women in centuries past, we seem to be more prone to osteoporosis than our female forebears. A team of researchers examining bones buried between 1729 and 1852 in the crypt of a London church found that the rate of bone deterioration was lower than in modern women of a similar age. They suggested that lack of exercise in modern lifestyles might be an important factor. The women buried in the crypt came from a section of the city dominated by the silk-weaving industry. Their work involved considerable movement in the upright position, activities now known to increase beneficial pressure on the skeleton and stimulation of bone formation.

To benefit bones, exercise has to be vigorous and prolonged, averaging three to five hours a week in total (adding together short bursts of activity) at 75 per cent of maximal aerobic capacity, that is, three-quarters of the peak workload that your heart and blood vessels can manage. And this workload has to be maintained. In one study, the benefit to bone density achieved during one year of an exercise program was lost entirely in the year after it finished.

Other inherited and lifestyle factors believed to contribute to osteoporosis include race (Asian and Caucasian women are at greater risk than Polynesian and Negroid women), a small body build, an excessive intake of alcohol or caffeine (from coffee, tea and soft drinks), insufficient dietary calcium, smoking, the intestinal malabsorption condition known as coeliac disease, a high salt intake, a diet rich in fat and protein, and the excessive use of antacids containing aluminium, or of cortisone-like drugs.

Mood-altering medications such as antidepressants, antipsychotics and benzodiazepines (for example, Clozapine and Diazepam) can also contribute to bone problems. Elderly patients taking these medications are more likely to have falls and fractures. The medications may add blood pressure changes and physical instability to existing vision problems, poor flexibility, and depleted muscle mass and strength.

As mentioned briefly, osteoporosis is more likely in women who have an early surgical removal of their ovaries, a hysterectomy without removal of the ovaries or a premature natural menopause (before the age of forty). In addition, you may be more likely to get osteoporosis if you have had anorexia nervosa, exercised so much at some time that your menstrual periods stopped for six or more months (known as amenorrhoea), used steroids over a long period (for example, to treat asthma or arthritis) or been confined to bed for some months, perhaps because of a serious accident.

Bobbi was in her early fifties when she fractured her wrist after slipping on some wet grass. Her medical history included a three-year period of anorexia nervosa in her twenties, together with smoking throughout her adult years, so a DEXA investigation was ordered. This revealed a worryingly low bone density, which prompted Bobbi to quit smoking, improve her diet and start treatment with HRT. A bone density measurement two years later indicated that the deterioration of Bobbi's bones had been arrested.

The most important factor of all in determining your risk of osteoporosis is the genes that control the way your body functions, and that may conspire with neglect of weight-bearing exercise, smoking, or a low calcium intake. If genetic vulnerability is combined with any other risk factor, the likelihood of osteoporosis multiplies. Attempts to put figures on these risks have proved controversial.

> ### THE OSTEOPOROSIS CHECK-LIST
>
> If you are concerned that osteoporosis is quietly eating away at your bones, you may gain reassurance or an incentive to make lifestyle changes by doing the following.
> - Check whether you have any inherited or lifestyle factors that may contribute to your risk of osteoporosis.
> - Recall whether you have ever fractured a bone, say in the forearm or wrist, when the pressure or force applied to that part of the body was minimal.
> - Ask someone to measure your height to see if it has decreased and to tell you if your back is becoming rounded.
> - Think through your experience of general aches and pains in the bones.

Having gone through a check-list like this, Joan's concerns about the state of her bones intensified. Although only fifty-three, she believed she had a full hand for osteoporosis: many years of eating disorders and dieting, a sedentary lifestyle, and a mother recovering from her second hip fracture. After discussing the situation with her doctor and having a bone density measurement that suggested a problem in the making, she revamped her lifestyle step by step. 'My doctor was reluctant to prescribe hormones because of a previous breast cancer, but started me on a gentle but regular exercise program. A year later I am doing things I wouldn't have dreamed of. Simple things, like walking to the local shops and post-box instead of driving. I feel hungrier and eat more, yet because I am exercising regularly I am not putting on weight. My enjoyment of life has definitely picked up.'

HORMONES USED FOR OSTEOPOROSIS To make a significant impact on the risk of osteoporosis, you will require HRT for at least ten years, ideally starting therapy within about two years of the last menstrual period. It does appear that the longer a woman remains on HRT, the stronger her bones. Another factor to consider, if you are a smoker taking oestrogen to avoid osteoporosis, is the importance of quitting because smoking reduces oestrogen's protective effect on bone.

Various studies show a 50 to 75 per cent reduction in the risk of fracture from osteoporosis after extended HRT. An adequate hormone dose is vital. The minimum daily oral dose of oestrogen required for prevention of bone loss is 0.625 mg of Premarin, 1.25 to 2.5 mg of Ogen, 2 to 4 mg of Progynova, or 0.02 mg of Estigyn. Some women prescribed HRT primarily for symptom control have more than an adequate dose to maintain their bone strength. In other cases, the prescribed dose is insufficient to prevent bone loss: some women have a low tolerance of hormones and are on the minimum, others smoke or have dietary imbalances that interfere with oestrogen uptake, and others again have such a fast rate of bone loss that even maximum hormone doses cannot keep pace.

For example, Premarin protects bones in most women at a dose of 0.625 mg daily, but studies tracking women's bone density over a number of years indicate that 15 per cent need twice this amount to gain protection. Yet other studies show that half this amount, as little as 0.3 mg of Premarin a day, is effective if combined with a daily intake of 1500 mg of calcium. Women whose menopause occurred many years previously may need to start at a lower hormone dose to minimise possible unwanted effects like breast tenderness. Dosage levels may then be increased gradually if prevention of bone weakness is a major reason for taking HRT.

Oestrogens can be used in pill, implant or skin patch form. If you still have your uterus you will need to take a progestogen as well to protect its lining from an increased risk of cancer. The chances of this cancer developing are about one in 25 000 for women before menopause, and one in 1100 for women not on oestrogen after menopause or women with a uterus receiving both oestrogen and progestogen. The risk of endometrial cancer for women with a uterus who use oestrogen alone in pill, patch or implant form for five years or more after menopause increases to approximately one in 200. However, with an adequate dose and duration of progestogen, the risk falls again to one in 1100 or less.

HRT AND ESTABLISHED OSTEOPOROSIS   Oestrogen therapy is effective in reducing bone loss even if given many years after menopause to women with osteoporosis. There is some evidence that it actually increases bone formation slightly, and that it may also reduce bone pain if this is a problem. Progestogens, testosterone and anabolic steroids (sometimes used to treat osteoporosis that causes debilitating pain in the spine) are also capable of preventing bone loss after menopause, but are not so widely used. The current evidence suggests that treatment with hormones will benefit women up to the age of at least seventy. Follow-up and monitoring, usually at intervals of six to twelve months, are essential to

In order to build an adequate peak bone mass through childhood and adolescence, four to five daily serves of calcium-rich food are necessary

check on side effects and to ensure that the therapy has effectively stopped bone loss.

HRT and heart or blood vessel disease

Premenopausal women have only one-fifth the risk of heart disease that men of the same age have. After menopause the gap closes, and a woman's risk of heart disease increases markedly, so that in the sixty to sixty-five age group heart disease risk in women is only one-third that of men. This change in risk is usually explained in terms of the decline in oestrogen levels after menopause.

Differences in stroke rates between women and men are not so pronounced. Women have approximately two-thirds the chance of stroke of men up to the age of sixty-five. The rates are similar for the over-seventies. Above eighty-five, when women well and truly overhaul men, numerically speaking, the absolute number of strokes in women is higher.

Overall, about half of all women in Australia die of heart or blood vessel diseases including stroke, and in women aged twenty to sixty-nine years there are an estimated 10 000 heart attacks a year.

One of Australia's leading heart research centres, the Baker Medical Research Institute in Melbourne, discussed the image and reality of heart and blood vessel disease in its 1992 Annual Report. 'When we think of cardiovascular disease, it tends to be in terms of heart attacks and cholesterol and blood pressure. When we think of how to prevent cardiovascular disease, it's things like diet and exercise and giving up cigarettes. And historically, we've thought about men and heart attacks; 85 per cent of heart transplants, for example, have had male recipients.

'The fact is that women are relatively protected, in terms of their cardiovascular status, by having oestrogens. It's relative because it's true as long as they have oestrogens. After the menopause, however, the incidence of heart disease rises rapidly, parallel to that in men; and as everybody knows, women live on average seven years longer. While men may have a head start, women have a higher chance of living widowed and with serious cardiovascular disease.'

Another unpalatable reality is that the causes and the most effective prevention and treatment strategies for heart disease in women are still being learned, whereas they are well established for men with heart disease. This discrepancy relates to the male focus of much heart disease research, a fact that concerns health authorities in many countries. 'Women die of heart disease almost as often as men do, but later in their lives,' says Judith Dwyer, who chairs the Women's Health Committee of Australia's major health watchdog, the National Health and Medical Research Council. 'It is surely inexcusable to base clinical advice on data that is good for the gander but may be worse than useless for the goose, even if that data is easier to gather.'

Judith Dwyer says the exclusion of women as participants in heart research is longstanding and ingrained in the system that governs trials of new pharmaceuticals. 'Drug companies in Australia are almost required to use only healthy, young male volunteers when testing new formulations,' she says. 'It seems to me to be perfectly possible to develop methods of avoiding many of the perceived problems, such as the danger of liability in the case of pregnancy in women.' In a bid to overcome the problem, a new approach has been devised to redress this kind of imbalance in Australian heart research.

FACTORS CONTRIBUTING TO HEART AND BLOOD VESSEL DISEASE   Given the lack of research on women and heart disease or stroke, questions arise as to the knowledge on which treatment strategies are based. What factors increase a woman's risk of having a heart attack or stroke? To what extent can we borrow from the heart research performed on men in devising prevention, diagnosis and treatment strategies?

Research that has examined these sorts of questions in women shows that your risk of developing a disease of the heart or blood vessels is higher than average if you have a family history of heart disease, blood clot disorders or strokes; had a hysterectomy before menopause (with or without removal of the ovaries); suffer from high blood pressure; have blood cholesterol that is above average; smoke cigarettes; have diabetes; do not exercise regularly; have a poor diet; or are overweight.

The reassuring thing is that three of the factors on the list – smoking, blood cholesterol and blood pressure – are said to account for as much as 60 per cent of your risk. And each of these factors can be influenced by the kinds of lifestyle changes described in chapter 6. Heart disease risks can decline quite rapidly for the ex-smoker, returning to levels similar to those of a non-smoker in about five years. A balanced diet can lead to a reduction in total cholesterol of about 10 to 15 per cent, which corresponds to a 20 to 30 per cent reduction in the risk of heart disease. In people with very high blood pressure the benefits of antihypertensive treatment are clear, since death rates among those who go untreated are very high.

HORMONES USED FOR HEART AND BLOOD VESSEL DISEASE   Hormone replacement therapy for postmenopausal women has won some advocates who regard it as a way to further reduce heart disease deaths, which have been

Oestrogen in pill form seems to have significant benefits for the heart and blood vessels

declining in Australia and much of the Western world since the 1960s. Studies of postmenopausal women prescribed oestrogen in pill form consistently show a significant reduction (by about 20 to 50 per cent) in the risk of heart disease for these women compared with women not taking oestrogen.

Knowledge of how this protective effect works is increasing, especially oestrogen's favourable impact on blood fats, including cholesterol, and its capacity to reduce heart disease risk by preventing the gradual build-up of fatty material inside blood vessel walls (known as atherosclerosis). It also seems to increase the width of the small blood vessels, enhancing blood flow and reducing the risk of clot formation and life-threatening blood vessel blockage.

Natural oestrogens in pill form seem to have greater benefits for the heart than oestrogen in other forms (implants, patches, vaginal creams and pessaries, for example), but the research is at an early stage. In addition, there are unanswered questions about dosage and duration of use.

The relationship between heart disease and the use of hormone preparations that combine oestrogen and progestogens is not conclusive. The studies performed to date have been short-term and confined in the main to women who are in good general health, are well educated and well off. No information is yet available regarding the long-term effects that these hormone combinations have on a woman's risk of developing heart attacks, strokes and blood clot disorders. There have been some encouraging animal studies that suggest that pairing these hormones does benefit the lining of blood vessels. However, a number of short-term studies on women suggest that progestogens in higher-than-HRT doses reduce the degree of benefit provided by oestrogen.

HRT AND EXISTING HEART OR BLOOD VESSEL DISEASE

There is strong evidence that oestrogen may protect women

with pre-existing heart and blood vessel disease from a further deterioration in their condition. There are also early indications that oestrogen reduces the tendency of major blood vessels to spasm in women prone to the excruciating heart pain, angina.

SUMMING UP THE POTENTIAL BENEFITS...

- The most identifiable short-term benefit is relief of symptoms such as hot flushes, night sweats and painful intercourse due to dryness of the vagina. Women with urinary symptoms of frequency and difficulty with bladder control may respond to HRT. Depression and sleeplessness occurring for the first time at menopause may also be relieved by HRT, and some women report improvements in memory, anxiety levels, uncharacteristic mood swings, interest in sex, and self-esteem.
- The most important established long-term benefit of hormone therapy is the prevention of bone loss, particularly of the hip, wrist and spine, and hence a reduction in the risk of fractures in elderly women. This effect has been shown with oestrogen and progestogen, but long-term studies with different formulations and combinations are incomplete.
- Long-term oestrogen therapy after menopause appears to reduce the risk of heart disease, particularly in women who already have it or are at high risk. Research is under way to determine whether combinations of hormones have the same effect. Definite answers are not expected for some years.

CHAPTER 4

The risks

THE HORMONES prescribed at and after menopause have powerful effects on many body systems. The very fact that they can dampen down hot flushes and night sweats in a matter of days, improve vaginal and urinary symptoms just as quickly, and change the course of heart disease and osteoporosis over a longer period is an indicator of their potency as well as the breadth of their impact. Unlike medications used in many other therapies, they do not have a narrow function. HRT affects many body systems, and it would be remiss of us to gloss over its downside or the uncertainties about it.

While HRT causes no major side effects in a majority of women, some others experience unwanted results that are totally unexpected. Sometimes women accept the risks of HRT because of an anticipated improvement in their quality of life in the immediate or distant future.

GAPS IN KNOWLEDGE   A problem with much of the

evidence about the benefits and risks of HRT is that the early research was into oestrogens alone, not the combination with progestogen. For women who don't have a uterus, and who therefore do not take a progestogen, this is not important. But the concern for the much larger number of women who take a combination of hormones is that the long-term effects on heart disease, blood vessel disorders and bone health are not known. There is still a great deal of prolonged research

Some women, fully informed about the risks of HRT, may accept them in anticipation of an improvement in their quality of life in the immediate or distant future

needed before we can tell women which progestogens are least disadvantageous, in what dose, and combined with what oestrogen.

Many studies show that women with a uterus who use oestrogen on its own for longer than six months experience an increased risk of cancer of the endometrium (lining of the uterus). By adding an adequate amount of progestogen for ten to fourteen days a month, we can make sure that the endometrium is protected.

Other concerns relevant to all women include the following.
- The apparent benefit of oestrogen in reducing the risk of heart disease may be due, partly at least, to bias in the selection of the women studied. All the studies of the risks and benefits of HRT are overshadowed by a big question mark. Are women who use it somehow different from the remainder of the female population, and if so might this skew the results? Are they healthier and at less risk of heart disease to

start with, for example? Are they more health-conscious at the outset? Are they careful about eating nutritious foods, not smoking, exercising regularly? And are they more likely to follow their doctor's suggestions? To be sure that HRT really benefits the heart it would be necessary to give HRT to one group of women selected from the general population and a placebo (a harmless and inert substitute) to a comparable group. The results of three such trials, which are at an early stage in the US, will be of interest.

- There is as yet only a limited amount of research evidence about short-term use of oestrogen patches, implants, vaginal creams and pessaries. No one knows yet whether the body handles oestrogen from these sources differently from oestrogen taken by mouth, or whether oestrogen in these forms offers protection against the development of heart

A concern for the large number of women who take progestogen as well as oestrogen at and after menopause is that the long-term effects on heart disease and blood vessel disorders are not known

and blood vessel disease. Preliminary data suggests that oestrogen administered in these ways produces beneficial changes to blood fat levels, and long-term findings are eagerly awaited from several studies capable of providing answers.

- It is still unclear to what extent cardiovascular disease and osteoporosis are due to oestrogen deficiency and to what extent they can be remedied by HRT.

- There is good evidence that heart disease risk factors for men, on whom most research has been done, cannot be applied holus-bolus to women. Since the risk of heart disease is figuring more and more among the reasons why doctors prescribe HRT, this raises questions about the basis on which such decisions are made.

> *The results of earlier studies of oestrogen cannot be assumed to apply today. These studies were conducted at a time when higher dosages and synthetic formulations of oestrogen were the norm*

- Menopause seems to have a range of effects on blood clotting factors and cholesterol, depending on how menopause came about. Even before women embark on HRT or bypass it, those who have had a surgical menopause are at greater risk of heart and blood vessel disease than women whose menopause occurred naturally. Many studies of HRT preparations have not taken account of this.
- Another problem with interpreting HRT studies is their frequent failure to separate dose and hormone type from duration of use. Although this information is sometimes hard to obtain, it is an important consideration because women who have been using oestrogen for a long time started it in an era when higher doses and synthetic formulations were more commonly prescribed. In short, the results of earlier studies of HRT cannot be assumed to apply today without taking account of the formulations and dosages used.
- Women on HRT are more likely to be examined by a

doctor and to have regular screening tests and monitoring of their general health than those who are not. This might result in a false picture of risks to health posed by HRT (because diseases not picked up in the general female population may be recognised in the HRT group as a result of their seeing doctors regularly and having more investigations). Paradoxically, the HRT group might survive longer, not necessarily because of any benefits conferred by their hormone treatment but because their routine monitoring might result in earlier disease detection, when the chances of successful treatment tend to be better.
- The current upsurge of interest in HRT is occurring at a time when heart disease rates are declining and breast cancer rates are increasing in countries like Australia and the US. HRT may be contributing to these trends, but the extent of this contribution is controversial.

HRT and the risk of developing breast cancer

The influence of hormone therapy on breast cancer risk is uncertain, despite numerous studies focused on this issue. The findings to date suggest the following.
- There is no increased risk of breast cancer from use of oestrogen for up to five years.
- For five to ten years of use a grey area exists, and any increase in breast cancer is probably below 30 per cent.
- For ten years or more of use, there may be a 30 to 80 per cent increase in the risk of breast cancer. This risk appears to be at the higher end of the range in women with a family history of breast cancer (including a mother, sister or daughter affected by the disease) and those using above-average doses of oestrogen (page 175 has average doses). Other risk factors for breast cancer are noted in chapter 7.

- It is unclear whether use of a progestogen in combination with oestrogen increases or decreases the risk of breast cancer. Dosages, and hormone types and methods, are not always documented fully in research studies, and this results in unnecessary ambiguity.
- Unanswered questions remain about whether breast cancer risk is increased by the use of oestrogen alone (in women with and without a uterus). There is also debate about whether progestogens teamed with oestrogen are more likely to reduce breast cancer risk if they are taken continuously or for ten to fourteen days a month, as described in chapter 2.

Because of these uncertainties it is very important, if you are on HRT, to be particularly careful to examine your own breasts regularly for any unusual lump or thickening, to have an annual examination of your breasts carried out by your doctor, and to have a mammogram every one to three years. Regular mammograms seem to be a particularly valuable safeguard.

HRT AND PREVIOUS BREAST CANCER Women with a previous breast cancer are usually advised against having HRT, although there are exceptions. Occasionally a woman

Women on HRT for longer than ten years seem to have an increased risk of developing breast cancer

whose breast cancer has been successfully treated, or who is having palliative care for breast cancer, may have such crippling menopausal symptoms that she decides to go onto HRT to get some relief.

Linda, for example, faced this dilemma when she developed

severe hot flushes in her late forties. She had been well for fifteen years following a mastectomy and, after discussions

✐ Have a mammogram every one to three years, do regular breast self-examination, and have your breasts checked by a doctor annually

with her breast specialist, decided to go ahead with HRT at the minimum dose needed to relieve her symptoms. Linda's doctor prescribed a natural oestrogen, similar to the oestradiol her ovaries had been secreting until not long before, and kept a close watch on all aspects of her health.

HRT and the risk of developing endometrial cancer

Women with a uterus who use oestrogen on its own for several years face a risk of endometrial cancer that is five to ten times greater than for women not using oestrogen at all. After more than ten years of use, the risk is more than ten times greater than might be expected. Even after oestrogen is no longer being taken, the risk persists for many years, if not decades. This is why many doctors are reluctant to prescribe oestrogen on its own (in pill, patch or implant form) to women with a uterus, preferring to add progestogen to protect the endometrium from possible cancer development. The most common exception is oestrogen in the form of vaginal creams, tablets and pessaries. These formulations can be used safely on their own provided that medical instructions are followed – daily for a week or so, but thereafter not more often than about two or three times a week.

Reassuringly, women who develop endometrial cancer while taking oestrogen typically have a good chance of survival. This is probably because doctors tend to keep a close watch on the health of such women and, at the first sign of unusual bleeding, the endometrium is examined and curative surgery performed.

HRT AND PREVIOUS ENDOMETRIAL CANCER Women with a recently treated endometrial cancer are generally advised not to have HRT. However, several years after successful treatment of early-stage endometrial cancer, hormone therapy incorporating both oestrogen and progestogen may be considered suitable.

Other disorders

The effects of oestrogen on the following disorders have been studied in some detail during the past fifty years. The impact of added progestogen is not so well understood.

HRT AND OVARIAN CANCER No consistent link has been demonstrated between HRT and ovarian cancer, but such a link has not been adequately ruled out. There is some evidence of ovarian cancer a substantial time after long-term HRT use. On the other hand, Pill-users (taking similar hormones to those of HRT but at higher doses) seem to be protected somewhat from ovarian cancer. Research in this area is continuing, but as yet no definitive conclusions can be drawn.

WOMEN WITH EXISTING LIVER DISEASE This condition becomes evident from abnormal liver function test results indicating that the liver is having difficulty doing its job of breaking down a wide range of substances. Recommendations regarding HRT for women with liver disease usually hinge on the nature and severity of the problem. In cases of severe active liver disease with abnormal liver function, HRT should be withheld. If the liver disease is mild or has resolved, HRT may be appropriate; in these cases the patch is the preferred way of administering it. This is because it is less demanding on the liver for absorption of hormones to be through the skin than via the stomach. While patches may be suitable for women with mild abnormalities of liver function, remember the reservation expressed at the beginning of this chapter about the lack of long-term research data on patches.

WOMEN WITH UNDIAGNOSED VAGINAL BLEEDING Until the reason for unexplained vaginal bleeding is diagnosed it is unwise for women to have HRT. The safest course of action is to have the bleeding investigated. This may entail a hysteroscopy and biopsy or curettage (see chapter 2).

WOMEN WITH HIGH BLOOD PRESSURE OR A HISTORY OF BLOOD CLOT TROUBLES Such women need more intensive surveillance than usual if they try HRT. In any case, it is a good idea for women on HRT to have their blood pressure checked regularly. If significant changes occur, it is important to have a full medical assessment and prompt treatment to control the problem (with blood pressure medications).

If you have a personal history of blood clots that developed for no apparent reason, or a family history of clotting disorders, you should tread cautiously where HRT is concerned. A thorough investigation of clotting function should be completed before deciding about whether or not to embark on hormone therapy. Genevieve developed a spontaneous clot in one leg during her thirties and, many years later, when she was contemplating HRT, a full investigation of her clotting factors was carried out. These revealed some minor abnormalities. However, Genevieve decided to start on a hormone patch to relieve her wide-ranging and severe menopausal symptoms. She asked her doctor about using aspirin to minimise the risk of further clot development, and was told that this was appropriate in her situation.

If clots are triggered by something definite like pregnancy, childbirth or previous surgery, HRT in patch form may be considered suitable. Some studies suggest that HRT does not significantly increase the risk of clots. But where there is any doubt it is wise to avoid taking the hormones in pill form, giving preference to patches. This is because the liver, which plays a major role in blood pressure control and blood clot formation, may become overactive when called on to handle the larger hormone load that occurs with pill formats (the patch releases hormones more gradually).

WOMEN WITH UTERINE FIBROIDS   Hormone replacement therapy does not cause problems with fibroids in most cases, but occasionally it results in heavy withdrawal bleeding. This calls for an investigation, to check where the fibroids are and what they are doing. If they are bulging into the cavity of the uterus, consideration may be given to removal of the endometrium by the technique described in chapter 7 (endometrial ablation). Fibroids generally shrink rapidly after menopause due to the reduction in overall oestrogen levels, or they may remain the same size. However, if you are on HRT your fibroids may shrink less quickly. High-dose oestrogen, especially in the form of implants, may produce significant growth in uterine fibroids, so you should avoid this way of taking it in.

Lorraine's experience of postmenopausal HRT included prolonged and heavy bleeding each month. Unusually, this persisted even after endometrial ablation. Her gynaecologist made a full assessment and gave Lorraine the option of stopping the HRT or, if she wanted to continue with it, to have a hysterectomy or a repeat ablation. She decided to withdraw from HRT and found her other major menopausal symptoms

– flushes, vaginal dryness, insomnia and mood swings – were becoming less distressing.

WOMEN WITH GALL BLADDER DISEASE Hormone replacement therapy undertaken by such women may change the composition of bile and increase the incidence of gallstones. If you have gallstones and want HRT, be cautious about it and give preference to the patch format. Hormone therapy is suitable for women who have had their gall bladders removed, provided there are no other reasons against it.

WOMEN WITH DIABETES Hormone replacement therapy may be prescribed for women with diabetes. However, if you have diabetes you should realise that your blood sugar levels are likely to be disrupted during the first few months of hormone use. This may necessitate changes in the dosage and timing of your medications, particularly if you use insulin. Patches or implants are the preferred form of HRT for women with diabetes. Although some research has been conducted on the impact of oestrogen on blood glucose levels, there is relatively little information on the effects produced by hormone combinations such as oestrogen and progestogen.

WOMEN WITH BENIGN BREAST LUMPS Most breast lumps are benign, and once they have been checked there is no special reason to avoid HRT. If examination of a lump shows any unusual cells or indicates that the growth of cells is abnormal, you are already at increased risk of breast cancer and the lump should be monitored carefully to pick up any change at an early stage. Regular monitoring of breast health by mammography, medical examination and self-examination of the breasts are vitally important.

WOMEN WITH ENDOMETRIOSIS This condition may be reactivated by oestrogen when treatment is started soon after menopause, especially if the menopause was surgical and the hormones are given in implant form. If a woman with endometriosis receives HRT, the patch or oral form of therapy is advisable. In theory the use of progestogen should help to keep the endometriosis under control in the first year after surgery, but this has yet to be confirmed.

Some unwanted effects of HRT

In addition to the possible interaction between HRT and existing medical conditions, there may be a range of unwanted symptoms caused by HRT itself. You may be bothered by one or other of the following.

BREAST TENDERNESS, FLUID RETENTION AND NAUSEA These symptoms are more likely in women who start on HRT some years after menopause. If nausea persists with the therapy in pill form, a different route should be considered, such as skin patches or implants. Breast tenderness often settles after a few months of HRT. If it persists, consideration should be given to a reduced dose of oestrogen, to a different way of administering it, and to complementary naturopathic remedies such as evening primrose oil tablets (see chapter 6).

WEIGHT GAIN About a quarter of women starting on HRT experience a small weight gain (up to 3 kg) during the first cycle and for a few months after. A smaller proportion put on considerable weight, part of which seems to be due to fluid retention. Some other women gain weight because of increased muscle mass – because they have discovered exercise in midlife. In older women who already have trouble moving freely, further weight can present problems because it makes regular activity more difficult.

Heather was sixty-eight when her doctor suggested she go onto HRT because of a personal and family history of heart disease. (She had already had coronary bypass surgery and her mother had died of a heart attack.) Heather's weight shot up after starting on a twice-weekly oestrogen patch and daily progestogen tablets. The doctor reduced the dose of the patch but her weight increase continued, amounting to 13 kg over a ten-month period. In consultation with her doctor she embarked on a program of exercise and dieting aimed at getting her weight down and benefiting her heart. At the time of writing she was trying to decide whether HRT was worth the trouble. 'I'm looking at the information and making up my mind whether to continue with HRT,' Heather said.

HEADACHE Nearly a third of women aged forty-five to fifty-five who participated in the Melbourne Women's Midlife Health Study complained of headaches. Given this prevalence, it is surprising how little research has been done on the relationship between headaches and hormones. For a small number of women, their first experience of headache seems to occur around the time of menopause, while for others they become less frequent. It is not known why this is so.

If you begin to have severe headaches, including migraine and visual or sensory disturbance, at about the time you start on HRT, you should stop and have the problem investigated. If you already had a headache problem and are on HRT, the situation should be watched closely. Be sure to check that your doctor is prescribing a 'natural' rather than a 'synthetic' oestrogen and a form of progestogen that is least likely to make headaches worse. Changing the brand of oral oestrogen or changing from a pill to a patch or implant may also help.

VAGINAL DISCHARGE Women can expect their normal vaginal lubrication to return while on HRT. Some women think they have developed a vaginal infection when it is simply a return of the natural mucus, which should make intercourse more comfortable.

WITHDRAWAL BLEEDS If you have a uterus you will

not necessarily experience withdrawal bleeds when you begin HRT. However, such bleeds (for a few days at a predictable time of the month) are more likely if progestogen is taken for ten to fourteen days a month along with daily oestrogen. In the case of a woman taking progestogen for the first twelve days each month, the withdrawal bleed typically starts between day twelve and day seventeen and occurs monthly. About half the women taking progestogen in this cyclical manner have withdrawal bleeds for ten years or more. In most cases the bleeds become progressively lighter. When HRT is discontinued, the bleeds stop.

Women taking progestogen each day in combination with oestrogen are less likely to have withdrawal bleeds as time goes by. Shirley was one of the 10 to 20 per cent of women using this format who have irregular spotting or bleeding six months to a year after starting. She found the irregular bleeding a nuisance but persisted with HRT because of a remarkable improvement in her vaginal symptoms and joint pain. Shirley's doctor suggested that continuation of the bleeding beyond twelve months should be investigated by endometrial biopsy or hysteroscopy and biopsy. By the time a year was up, all bleeding had stopped.

Whether you take progestogen for a part or all of a cycle, the first few withdrawal bleeds are likely to be the heaviest, particularly if you start on HRT around the time of menopause. At this stage there may be some endometrium left, and the initial courses of progestogen produce the first bleeds after several months of build-up.

Heavy withdrawal bleeding generally responds to an increase in the dosage or potency of the progestogen used to balance the oestrogen. If bleeding continues despite alterations in dosage, it suggests the presence of uterine fibroids or endometrial polyps. These should be investigated by hysteroscopy and biopsy, and may be removed subsequently along with most of the endometrium by techniques including endometrial ablation (see chapter 7). Even after this therapy, women need to keep taking progestogen as it is impossible to remove all of the endometrium.

Women who do not start HRT until several years after the menopause usually have less endometrium than those at, or with a recently completed, menopause. If you are older than that, the amount of endometrium may be insufficient to produce any visible withdrawal bleed. The absence of a withdrawal bleed indicates that there is little endometrium to be shed.

BREAKTHROUGH BLEEDING Unexpected bleeding, known as breakthrough bleeding, can occur at any time of the month if you are taking both oestrogen and progestogen throughout your cycle. If you are on progestogen for only part of the cycle it can occur at times other than the end of the progestogen phase, and in such cases a thorough assessment by hysteroscopy is essential. If there is no problem with the endometrium, the dose of hormones is probably inadequate. The bleeding is usually stopped by alterations to the dose or potency of the oestrogen or progestogen.

If you do not want to have to cope with any bleeding, a change to the combined oestrogen and progestogen regimen may reduce breakthrough bleeding, or else you may consider having your endometrium removed. Paradoxically, although fewer women experience withdrawal bleeds with the combined format, about 10 per cent are still experiencing breakthrough bleeding a year later. The problem of breakthrough bleeding appears to be worse in women who are close to menopause or who have a recent history of disturbed bleeding, and it is for this reason that they are more likely to be given progestogen for part of the cycle rather than throughout it. Older women who are commencing HRT after several years without a bleed seem to have fewer problems with breakthrough bleeding.

IRRITABILITY AND MOODINESS   A common short-term side effect of the progestogen component of HRT is irritability and moodiness reminiscent of the symptoms of premenstrual syndrome. Sometimes these side effects last longer, and very occasionally they persist despite trying various progestogens. If you are affected in this way, you may elect to stop HRT, or take oestrogen alone — accepting that hysteroscopy and biopsy will be necessary every six to twelve months.

SKIN REACTIONS   Occasionally menopausal women who use oestrogen develop a skin disorder called chloasma when exposed to the sun. The development of patches of darker skin on the face, legs and hands is similar to the skin reaction that sometimes occurs during pregnancy. The cause of the problem is uncertain, but deposits of melanin in the skin are involved. The discoloration usually becomes less noticeable when oestrogen therapy ceases, but it may become more noticeable on exposure to the sun, even after stopping HRT. Wearing a hat and applying a maximum-protection sunscreen should become part of your outdoor routine. Your doctor may have some suggestions about the most appropriate sunscreen in your particular case, and forms of treatment that may remove the discoloration.

Skin irritation or rash can occur when hormone patches are used and, less commonly, women report a more generalised allergic response. As we saw in the case of Margaret in chapter 1, this can be severe enough to cause the abandonment of patch therapy. The problem appears to be worse in hot climates, and the reported incidence varies from 5 to 40 per cent in user groups worldwide. Occasionally there is also a severe local allergic response to the patch adhesive.

SUMMING UP THE POTENTIAL RISKS . . .

- There are still many uncertainties about the long-term impact of HRT on body tissues. Research is under way, but definite answers will not be available until around the year 2000.
- Breast cancer risk may be increased by 30 to 80 per cent in women using HRT for ten years or more. If such a risk does occur (and this is controversial), their risk would rise to about one in ten, compared with about one in fourteen for similar women who do not use HRT. Women whose risk is at the higher end of the range are those who have a strong family history of breast cancer, a previous breast cancer, or abnormal cells in a breast biopsy.
- The risk of endometrial cancer is five to ten times higher for women with a uterus taking oestrogen alone for more than five years, compared with similar women not on HRT. This increased risk does not apply where vaginal oestrogen is used according to medical instructions, or when adequate oestrogen and progestogen are used by women with a uterus.
- There is a slight increase in gall bladder disease.
- Uterine fibroids and, rarely, endometriosis may bleed heavily with HRT, especially in women on implants.
- Breakthrough bleeding is a common problem with some regimens of HRT.
- Nausea, breast tenderness, weight gain and skin reactions may also occur, necessitating a change in dosage or in the way the hormone is given.

CHAPTER 5
....

You and your sex life

*I*T HAS TRADITIONALLY been assumed that women at and after the menopause are likely to lose interest in sex – that sexual desire ebbs from the forties onwards and drifts relentlessly downwards. Older women who have an evident – perhaps even a lusty – interest in sex tend to be caricatured as clinging pathetically to lost youth, being somehow depraved, or as having 'emotional' problems. The American writer Dorothy Parker put the whole matter on a cheery footing in her poem 'The Little Old Lady in Lavender Silk'. At 'seventy-seven, come August' she had faced up to the 'passing from Summer to Fall' and believed that, throughout her long life, there was 'nothing more fun than a man'. These sentiments are echoed in recent careful reviews of medical and social research that paint a different, more complex picture of sexual activity after menopause.

Numerous studies show no clear evidence of a consistent

and predictable decline in sexual desire or activity among older women. Rather there is wide variability, with the presence of a suitable male partner being more important than age. Edward Brecher's 1984 study of sexuality and ageing, the largest since Alfred Kinsey's study of 1938, found a clear decline in sexual activity among US women over the age of fifty compared with men. But when he took account of whether the women were married or widowed (that is, presumably deprived of easy access to a partner), he found almost identical levels of sexual activity for both sexes.

Other studies, such as that of Dr Gloria Bachmann, suggest that sexual activity may decline if problems such as lubrication are not dealt with; if night sweats and insomnia are severe and persistent; if either partner is ill; if the male partner has a medical problem or takes medication that affects his sexual capability; if partners are unhappy in their relationship; or if they are subject to other major life stresses. Perhaps such factors help to explain the finding of the Melbourne Women's Midlife Health Study that nearly a third of women who had a natural menopause between the ages of forty-five and fifty-five reported a decline in sexual interest.

Cultural values and traditions may also have subtle influences on sexual activity. For example, if sex is valued mainly for the children that may result, sexual activity may be restricted to the fertile years. On the other hand, in societies that value sexuality in older women and do not consider that female attractiveness resides solely with the young, post-menopausal women are more likely to be sexually active.

> *Libido is not merely a matter of hormones. What is in your head and heart will also affect your interest in sex*

So it is clear that there is little to suggest, among women with suitable opportunities, an inevitable or precipitous fall in sexual activity at or after menopause.

Differing views

When Libby Hathorn and Glenn Bates interviewed more than 130 Australian men and women aged up to fifty-five for their book *Half-Time*, they commented on the diversity of views that women participants held on sex. Regardless of whether they had reached menopause or not, some women found sex disappointing, and less enjoyable as they got older: it wasn't fulfilling; it had become mechanical, lacked excitement and adventure; or their partner was insensitive to their needs and feelings. The opportunity to reduce or discontinue sexual activities under the socially acceptable excuse of 'sexless middle age' was for some a great relief. However, most felt that with age came greater self-confidence, less anxiety, a deep satisfaction in their sexual relations, and a greater enjoyment of cuddling and shared sexual intimacies than they had ever thought possible.

Women who had reached menopause also had varied views on sex. Some had lost interest in it and were not concerned at seeing it lose some of its significance in their lives, while others were taking more initiative in sexual relations. Though women said they needed to have more direct stimulation to get aroused during sex, and orgasms were less frequent for some, they still felt a strong sexual drive and found the total sexual experience very pleasurable.

Feedback from women about their experiences of sex at and after menopause confirms this range of views. Some, such as Betty, who fell in love with a younger man while in her fifties, view sex as a crucial part of the relationship. 'I feel good about myself and about my partner, and wonderful sex seems to flow from that. Since I'm no beauty, I've always tried to make sure I'm interesting company: this means spending time regularly on activities that extend my interests and challenge me. My partner and I are very conscious of looking our best for each other, and so eating healthy foods and taking regular exercise have become part of our life together.'

Others we spoke to had found new opportunities for romance, triggered by a change of partner, a variation or development in the relationship with their existing partner, a greater acceptance of themselves, or simply a freedom from anxieties about contraception and pregnancy. Other couples had compensated for joyless sex by developing satisfying non-sexual

> *Numerous studies show no clear evidence of a consistent and predictable decline in sexual desire or activity among older women. Rather there is wide variability, with the presence of a suitable male partner being more important than age*

activities, or else sex had been relegated to the background because one or other partner felt overwhelmed by problems associated with dependent children, dependent parents or in-laws, or financial burdens.

June's life is full of pressures from which sex provides no release. She has effectively vetoed sex with her husband, declaring her unwillingness to put any more energy into it. In doing so, she admits that she is also making a statement about her dissatisfaction with her husband for letting himself 'go to seed'.

There are other couples who have put intimacy on hold, pending treatment for a disability or serious illness. The partner who is in good health sometimes admits to mixed feelings: anger or irritation that his or her sexual needs cannot be satisfied within the relationship, and guilt for lacking compassion over a partner's ill health. Ailing partners may also feel distressed about their inability to participate in an active sex life.

This was the case until a few years ago for Emily, a sixty-two-year-old who suffered from chronic back pain. Initially she was very concerned to protect her back, and she put sex off limits. But with support and reassurance from various health practitioners, she experimented and found enjoyable ways to have sex with her partner. In particular, she chose times when she was warm, well rested and feeling sexy, and with plenty of pillows available to support her back.

For Nadia, who was plagued by intermittent heavy bleeding in her mid-forties, the problem was finding a time when she could have sex enjoyably. 'I had never felt like sex during my monthly bleeds, but at least they previously lasted only four or five days. This stage was much worse because I was bleeding for fifteen days without a break and I felt so ugh! My husband didn't mind having sex while I was bleeding, but I just couldn't come at it.' Since Nadia's menopause at the age of forty-eight, she and her husband have resumed the satisfying sex life they enjoyed in earlier years.

Sexuality and emotional growth

Sex is not a precondition for a happy and satisfying life. If sex is not part of a relationship, lack of interest in it is a matter of concern only if it becomes personally troubling or causes problems in relating to others. It cannot be said too strongly that those who have neither a desire for nor interest in sex, or who have deliberately chosen a lifestyle in which sexual activities play little or no part, have every right to their decision. On the other hand, those older people who enjoy sex or want to enjoy it should be given the information and treatment they need if problems arise.

In attempting to put the presence or absence of sexual intimacy into some sort of general framework of midlife relationships, Hathorn and Bates identified a significant obstacle. 'One of the major problems was that our interest was in both men and women, yet it seems that most of the well-known developmental theorists of the past have focused only on men. It is as if woman were an afterthought and had to be "fitted in" to men's cycle of growth.'

Professor Marjorie Fiske, who initiated a long-term study of life changes among Californian adults, believes that developmental models based on men may be misleading where women are concerned. 'The assumption that men and women undergo similar processes in terms of developing, coping, and "declining" has turned out to be fallacious. In nearly all ways of living, thinking and feeling, a young woman is far more likely to resemble an older woman than a young man her own age. Similarly, differences between groups of men in various periods of life are less significant than their differences from women in their own life stage.'

While women within male–female relationships have been largely overlooked by theorists, homosexual women and heterosexual women without partners have fared even worse, having had almost no attention paid to them in traditional analyses of sexuality after menopause. Simone de Beauvoir made the point in her book *The Coming of Age* that enjoyment of sexual activities takes many forms, has many motivations, and is not necessarily extinguished with age. 'It is understandable that a man or woman should be bitterly unwilling to give it up, whether the chief aim is pleasure, or the transfiguration of the world by desire, or the realisation of a certain image of oneself, or all this at the same time . . . The old person often desires to desire because she retains her longing for experiences that can never be replaced and because she is still attached to the erotic world she built up in her youth or maturity – desire will enable her to renew its fading colours.'

Menopausal symptoms and their impact on sexual feelings and intimacy

Discussions on sex after menopause tend to focus on one aspect above all others – the physical changes to the vaginal lining, which becomes thinner, less acidic, and more easily damaged with age. A compelling argument against this focus, put forward by Germaine Greer in *The Change*, is that 'it has been proved time and time again that women's orgasms do not originate in the vagina and that other forms of love play are more effective in pleasuring women . . . if she is one of the many women who have been fucked when they wanted to be cuddled, given sex when what they really wanted was tenderness and affection, the prospect of more of the same until death do her part from it is hardly something to cheer about.' Granted the truth of this, there may be times when vaginal sex or masturbation is sought by women, in which case it is not much fun feeling as dry as the Nullarbor and being about as responsive as a derailed train. Finding the oasis in the desert can be a struggle, though HRT can be very helpful.

Christine was incensed by some friendly advice to 'use it or lose it' when she related that sex with her husband was unsatisfactory. 'How can I use it when it feels like scratching an open wound?' she asked. Once she had faced the need for alternative sources of lubrication, and the vaginal lining became more elastic under the influence of oestrogen cream, a localised form of HRT prescribed by her doctor, Christine lost her fear that sex would hurt, and she started enjoying it again. 'All I need for good health and a long life is vegetables, fish, laughter and sex, not necessarily in that order,' she quipped.

Other physical aspects of menopause that can unsettle the desire for sexual intimacy involve changes in skin sensation. Barbara noticed a heightened sensitivity to touch soon after her menopause and literally could not bear the feeling of her nipples being stroked or her clitoris being stimulated, previously pleasurable sensations. 'I explained this to my husband so he didn't take it personally, and we agreed it would be a good idea if I discussed it with my doctor. She was very reassuring, explaining that the changing balance of hormones around menopause can have an effect on the sensitive nerve endings in the skin of some women, and that the altered sensation usually passes with time.'

How to improve sex during and after menopause

TAKE YOUR TIME   Four-minute sex is out. Spending time over love-making can enhance the experience for both you and your partner. Your natural lubrication needs a chance to develop, and men also tend to require more time to reach climax as they get older.

LUBRICATION AND OTHER AIDS   Vaginal lubricating compounds such as K-Y jelly, and new hormone-free substances that last for several days and are not messy (such as Replens), are helpful. You can also make use of 'male dew', the natural lubricant from the tip of the penis. Masturbation, either alone or with your partner, can also help to promote lubrication. Although frowned on in some religious circles, masturbation is widely regarded as a healthy way to handle sexual needs and expression with or without a partner. Some couples find that a hand-held vibrator and sexually stimulating magazines or videos also help. Think about your range of sexual positions. Be adventurous in trying new ones, bearing in mind that some will put less stress on vaginal tissues that would otherwise tend to be hurt by penetration. A woman on top, for example, has increased control of the situation. She should also take plenty of initiative in the type and duration of love-making and ensure that she is completely comfortable throughout.

TALK ABOUT IT   Don't assume that your partner understands what is going on inside your body or mind. Try

Four-minute sex is out. Spending time over love-making can enhance the experience for both you and your partner. Your natural lubrication needs a chance to develop, and men also tend to require more time to reach climax as they get older

to describe what you are experiencing – otherwise a partner may misinterpret your reluctance to have sex. It may also be desirable to arrange a consultation for both of you with a doctor or counsellor, to discuss your sexual concerns and possible approaches to overcoming them. If this is impossible, talk about your feelings with a friend, a sympathetic doctor or a counsellor.

LIBIDO   There are many documented cases of libido disappearing entirely in older people, men as well as women.

It seemed to George Bernard Shaw that, when he lost interest in women, he lost interest in living. 'I am ageing very quickly. I have lost all interest in women, and the interest they have in me is greater than ever and it bores me. The time has probably come for me to die.' If your lack of interest in sex concerns you, see your local doctor or an experienced counsellor. Alternatively, you could telephone your nearest Marriage

Women should use HRT to meet their own needs rather than those of others

Guidance Council office, the state office of the Australian Medical Association or the Australian Psychological Society and ask for the names of people who specialise in this field. If loss of interest in sex is not worrying you or disturbing your relationships with others, there is no need to take any action.

HORMONE THERAPY   The idea of prescribing HRT for women solely to keep them receptive to their partners' advances is outrageous, as Germaine Greer has argued. Unfortunately this seems to have happened in the 1970s. 'Because they desire the preservation of cosmetic youth and the unflagging libido of patients, physicians have championed estrogen [oestrogen] replacement therapy in the hope of attaining a maximal quality of life for their patients,' the US medical researchers Dr Harry Ziel and Dr William Finkle said in 1976. Equally objectionable were the pharmaceutical advertisements of this era that promoted HRT 'for the menopausal problems that bother *him* the most [our emphasis]'.

Yet there are many middle-aged and older women wanting to have genital sex with partners who feel the same. If the way their vaginas feel prevents this, they should consider the use of substances including oestrogen, either as a cream, tablet or pessary applied directly to the vagina, as pills to be swallowed, or in some other form. The crucial difference is that they understand and accept the therapy, with all its pros and cons, and use it to meet their own needs rather than the needs of others.

If you are wondering whether the direct application of oestrogen to the vagina has identical effects to that of oestrogen by pill, patch or implant, the answer is a conditional yes. Oestrogen-containing vaginal creams have the disadvantage of being messy, but they do increase lubrication and vaginal tone, and they may improve libido and feelings of wellbeing. They also impinge minimally on other body tissues when used as directed, thus reducing the chances of unwanted effects.

Testosterone implants to increase energy and sexual appetite are an appropriate option for some women. These can be used on their own or in addition to oestrogen.

SUPPORTIVE RELATIONSHIPS Psychological factors such as self-confidence, self-esteem and trust are intimately involved in the achievement of satisfying sex for both partners. Men are under greater pressure than women when it comes to sexual performance, and their capacity to have an erection and therefore penetrative sex may be reduced with age. Beyond the age of fifty or so, men generally require more stimulation than in their younger days to get an erection and to maintain it, reaching orgasm takes longer, and ejaculation may be more difficult. Penile sensation also tends to change.

According to Simone de Beauvoir, 'Whereas a man of a certain age is no longer capable of erection, a woman at no matter what age is endowed with as it were a furnace . . . all fire and fuel within'. Popular Scottish songs of the eighteenth century make much of this contrast. An elderly woman yearns for the wild embraces of her younger days, now no more than a ghostly memory, since her husband no longer thinks of doing anything in bed except sleep, while she is eaten up with desire.

As with most men, a woman's attitude to her physical appearance influences the way she relates sexually. Some studies indicate that men are even more concerned than women about the effects of ageing on their sexual desirability. As hair turns grey, with wrinkles becoming more prominent and bodies losing muscle tone, both men and women may see themselves as less attractive and less sexually desirable. If they cannot accept that an elderly person can also be beautiful, they may shy away from sexual intimacy.

It's worth remembering the personal traits that are independent of age – character, intelligence, expressiveness, warmth and personal style. These form the real basis of deep and lasting sexual attraction.

CHAPTER 6

Alternatives to HRT

WHO WOULD have believed, a generation ago, the current popularity of 'alternative' therapies and the challenge they have thrown down to orthodox medicine? There was little to indicate in the 1970s that the so-called fringe therapies like naturopathy, homeopathy, traditional Chinese medicine and herbal medicine would attract a vast pool of clients who alternated between orthodox and less conventional practitioners with breezy savoir-faire.

Equally unexpected were the greening of the Western diet and the enthusiastic adoption of power walking, jogging, aerobics and weight training by women of all ages. Many older women took to the challenge with gusto, viewing their increased involvement in physical activity as an antidote to the lack of strenuous exercise in their lives. When the 1991 Bulletin/Qantas Businesswoman of the Year, Sara Henderson, was writing her bestselling autobiography *From Strength to*

Strength and its sequel (still to be published at the time of writing), she felt the need to restructure her writing days to include short time-outs for exercise.

'I'd played sport till I was forty-five, mainly tennis and squash. And there was a lot of physical activity at Bullo, down in the yards, working gates, building fences, lifting cases of beer in and out of the store. [Sara and her daughters own and run Bullo River, a remote Northern Territory cattle station.] To keep in nick when I'm writing twelve hours a day, I take a few minutes off every hour or so and do a couple of hundred skips. In the evenings I walk some kilometres along the airstrip with the dogs and, before going to bed, I do weights for my upper body for twenty minutes or so.'

Sara went through a fairly straightforward menopause when she was fifty. There were several months of irregular and heavy bleeding, followed by a return to normal periods, then irregularity again and so on, the whole process taking about three years and coinciding with the deaths of her husband, mother and son-in-law. Sara has not had HRT, says that people comment on how well she looks, and remarks on how well she feels. She enjoys a balanced diet mainly of fresh meat, vegetables and fish, does not smoke, and since the age of forty-five has drunk alcohol on special occasions only.

Whether women choose HRT or not, they should be aware of the range of lifestyle changes and alternative or complementary therapies capable of lessening menopausal symptoms and enhancing long-term health.

A common criticism of alternative therapies is the lack of solid scientific evidence about their effectiveness and safety, a problem compounded by the lack of quality control in the manufacture of some substances. As with HRT, uncertainties about effects should be considered carefully in assessing the benefits and risks.

Hot flushes

Training in biofeedback and relaxation can play a valuable role in increasing a woman's ability to control her hot flushes. Biofeedback techniques teach people to manipulate particular body functions once thought to be independent of conscious control, for example heart rate, muscle tension, and the degree to which blood vessels in the skin open and close. In a typical biofeedback training program, a person who suffers severe headaches has an electronic instrument capable of measuring muscle tension attached to his or her forehead. The machine transforms this state into a beep or flashing light so that awareness grows of tensing up. With time and practice, the ability to self-monitor and control muscle tension increases.

Marie was one of a small number of women with debilitating flushes who took part in a biofeedback training program for a total of eight hours over a four-week period. Her experience was of a marked drop in hot flush activity and associated

> *Alternative therapies are often criticised for lack of solid scientific evidence, but even HRT needs more research*

discomfort. For the first time she felt able to 'short-circuit' at least some of her hot flushes by putting her biofeedback training into action at the first sign of a flush.

Relaxation training, yoga, regular acupuncture and meditation also seem capable of reducing hot flush frequency, especially when combined with other coping strategies, like wearing clothes in layers, choosing fabrics that 'breathe', and steering clear of neck-hugging dresses and blouses.

Non-hormonal prescription – as distinct from alternative – medications studied as treatments for hot flushes include propanolol (a treatment for angina and abnormal heartbeat, trade name Inderal), clonidine (a blood pressure medication, trade name Dixarit) and naproxen (a treatment for rheumatoid arthritis, trade name Naprosyn). These suffer from the disadvantage of not being as consistently effective in reducing flush

Vitamin E in supplement form should be used with caution and monitored regularly because it can interfere with normal blood clotting and may raise blood pressure

activity as hormonal therapies and, like most medications, they have undesirable side effects in some women. Sedatives and tranquillisers are sometimes prescribed for hot flushes and anxiety, but these may worsen other menopausal symptoms like lack of energy, and increase the likelihood of falls and fractures.

Herbs often used for hot flushes include *Cimicifuga racemosa*, which is said to have a direct action in reducing FSH levels (which relate to oestrogen levels – see page 171), plus ginseng, motherwort and lime blossom (taken in tincture form first thing in the morning and last thing at night). Ginseng is the common name of several species of *Panax* herbs, and it has been prized in the East for thousands of years. Modern research has confirmed that it reduces sweating and helps the body adapt to heat stress, enhancing energy and stamina in trying conditions. Ginseng comes in a wide variety of formulations, and we recommend a cautious approach to its use as excessive amounts can lead to high blood pressure and palpitations. If no improvement is seen with any herbal substance within four weeks, it is wise not to persist.

Vitamin E and evening primrose oil tablets have strong advocates among some women with severe flushes. Natural dietary sources of vitamin E are oils made from corn, soybeans,

> *Attending a gym in the evenings or having a brisk after-dinner walk can have a dramatic effect on insomnia by reducing the time needed for falling asleep*

coconut, peanuts and olives, plus alfalfa, barley, peanuts, rolled oats, chocolate, cabbage, spinach and asparagus. Vitamin E in supplement form should be used with caution and monitored regularly because it can interfere with normal blood clotting and raise blood pressure. As with all vitamins, it is preferable not to overdo the amount of vitamin E coming from supplements, and expert advice should be sought on dosage levels.

Regular physical activity is sometimes advocated for hot flush relief. The findings of the Melbourne Women's Midlife Health Study supported an association between exercise levels and feelings of good health when activities took participants outside the home. There was no apparent association, however, between exercise levels and the intensity and number of hot flushes experienced.

Headaches

Biofeedback training has been used with some success in patients with migraine headaches. Migraines around menopause have also been treated with the prescription medication clonidine, in lower doses than when it is used to treat blood pressure problems. The results of studies to assess symptom relief have been conflicting, and side effects may include dizzy spells, visual disturbances, and – astonishingly – headaches.

Sleeplessness

Calcium seems to help overcome sleeplessness, as do the popular herbal sedatives camomile tea and valerian root. Another 'therapy' for sleep disturbance that does not require 'taking' anything is physical activity. Attending a gym in the evenings or having a brisk after-dinner walk can have a dramatic effect on insomnia by reducing the time needed for falling asleep. Swimming releases excess energy that might otherwise cause tension, preparing the mind and body for sleep. Sex is also recommended.

Hints on increasing the likelihood of sleeping well and rising refreshed include the following.

- Spend some time, before you turn in, doing whatever relaxes you – listening to music, taking a warm bath, reading a book.
- Establish a simple routine every night before going to bed, even just having a shower and cleaning your teeth.
- Reduce or avoid alcohol, coffee and tea with your evening meal.
- Concentrate on relaxing every part of your body in stages as you lie in bed, from the tips of your toes to your forehead.
- Above all, don't worry about the amount of sleep you are getting – it is surprising how little one can survive on. A good night's sleep is whatever is normal for you, with some people requiring only a couple of hours.

Anxiety

One of the most distressing of the emotions reported by women at menopause is anxiety, which is often described as a feeling of impending doom. In the case of Joan, anxiety attacks became so severe around the time of her menopause that she withdrew from most of her former activities outside the home. Her state of anxiety was reduced markedly by a program of vigorous physical activity (exercising to loud music), which she started in her own home before joining the aerobics class at her local recreation centre.

Evening primrose oil tablets, St John's wort, oatstraw and *Anemone pulsatilla* are often advocated by herbal therapists and naturopaths for women disturbed by anxiety and panic attacks. You will need to consult such therapists for dosages.

Dry vagina and urinary symptoms

Vitamin A in tablet form is considered by many naturopaths to be useful in treating vaginal dryness and bladder irritability. The usual recommendation is to take it for six to eight weeks and then to have a two-week break. Alternatively they may recommend a vaginal ointment made from English marigolds (*Calendula officinalis*). This is credited with oestrogen-like properties and an ability to prevent and treat vaginal infections.

The pelvic floor muscles are like a safety net supporting all the organs of the lower abdomen. When the muscles are weak, any form of stress exerted on the bladder – such as a sudden jump, cough, laugh or lifting motion – can result in an outflow of urine. Increasing numbers of women are taught pelvic floor (Kegel) exercises, which they are encouraged to do daily. These exercises are designed to strengthen the

> **KEGEL EXERCISES**
>
> Locate your sphincter muscle (it controls urination) simply by stopping the urine flow; this means you are contracting your sphincter muscle. Practise a few times, stopping and starting the flow of urine at will.
>
> - Stop the flow of urine for three full seconds, then release for one second. Repeat six times, three times daily for a few days, then more often if time permits. With practice, you will not need to be urinating to know when you are contracting your sphincter muscle.
>
> *or*
>
> - Contract your sphincter muscle strongly for one second and release for one second. Speed up the contractions so that you experience a 'fluttering' feeling.
>
> *or*
>
> - Contract the muscle for ten full seconds then relax for five. Repeat five times, three times a day.

muscles that support the bladder, uterus and bowel, in order to control stress incontinence and prolapse. You can alternate the exercises and use triggers, such as stops at red traffic lights or brushing your teeth, to remind you to do them.

Lack of energy, feeling 'blue' or out of sorts

Strange as it may seem, feelings of lethargy are often associated with a lack of strenuous physical activity. Lack of exercise, especially exercise that takes you beyond your home, can make you feel rather depressed too. A program of regular moderate physical activity is one of the first things to consider when feeling out of sorts. In general, it is best to set a manageable target, beginning slowly and increasing the level of activity progressively. Inertia is one of the most difficult states to overcome. Setting too high a target can be counterproductive and may send you backwards.

Sticking to an exercise plan for a couple of weeks does wonders for morale and, instead of inventing excuses to avoid exercise, you will find it becomes something to look forward to with pleasure. In working out an exercise plan, there are some important factors to consider.

- The aim is to make regular physical activity part of your life, so choose something you enjoy – something that is convenient, interesting, can be done independently and is realistically achievable.
- If you are over forty or have high blood pressure, diabetes or a known heart problem, check with your doctor before you start your plan. A preliminary health check is sometimes advisable anyway, especially if you intend working up to strenuous forms of activity.
- Always warm up for at least five minutes before exercising, and cool down after it. Include some stretching exercises in the warm-up to reduce the risk of muscle strains.
- Never exercise if you are not feeling well. If illness interrupts your plan, resume at a lower level than before and slowly build up again.
- Tell your doctor about any symptoms you experience during exercise, particularly chest discomfort or undue dizziness.

Any woman at midlife who smokes should consider giving it away. If you are a typical twenty-cigarettes-a-day smoker who quits, you will experience changes something like these:

- Between twelve and twenty-four hours after stopping, you will start to feel less short of breath when you exert yourself.
- Within a couple of days you will begin to feel and smell fresher. Your taste buds will come alive and your sense of smell will return.
- Within three weeks your lungs will be working better and physical activity will be easier.
- Within two months, blood flow to your limbs will improve and you will have more energy.

If you have tried quitting repeatedly without success it may be time to consider a Quit group, which will provide a sound educational approach and ongoing support.

Finally, help for lethargy and depressed moods may be obtained from plants that contain oestrogen-like substances, called phyto-oestrogens. They seem to have less powerful effects than the oestrogens used in HRT, but are worth trying. Plants with a considerable amount of oestrogen-like content include alfalfa, aniseed, basil, caraway, chervil, the common beans, fennel, fenugreek, hops, licorice (which should be avoided by people with blood pressure problems), parsley, red clover, sage and soya bean sprouts.

Foods containing smaller amounts of oestrogen include fresh corn, corn oil, green peas, cabbage, wheat bran and wheat germ, rice bran and milk. The list is so long that you should have no difficulty finding something you can add to salad, vegetable or other dishes each day.

Bone health

Bone is a living substance and, like tissues such as the skin, it is constantly being removed and replaced. Normally this process is in balance, with the amount of old bone removed being replaced by an equal amount of freshly formed bone. To keep this balance it seems that bones need mechanical stress (the harder they have to work against the force of gravity, the stronger they get), together with a dietary supply of calcium, phosphorous, and tiny amounts of various other nutrients.

The types of exercise that seem most beneficial for bone strength are the weightbearing ones, such as walking, dancing, jogging, lawn bowls, gardening, golf and tennis. Associated benefits are an increase in flexibility and an opportunity for mixing with other people. How you feel during exercise is an important guide. Try to maintain a feeling of being a little 'pushed' without moving to the breathless stage.

Australian health authorities say that women at and after menopause need an estimated 1000 to 1500 mg of calcium a day to be in calcium balance. The Melbourne Women's Midlife Health Study indicates that only 5 per cent of women aged between forty-five and fifty-five have sufficient calcium in their diet to meet this recommendation. The study found that about 20 per cent of women get about 250 mg of calcium a day, a quarter of the recommended daily intake, and another 35 per cent have a calcium intake of less than 500 mg.

Eating foods rich in calcium or taking calcium supplements each day can bring calcium intake up to recommended levels. Foods rich in calcium include milk, tofu, cheese, soy milk, yoghurt, green vegetables, parsley, cabbage, seaweed, almonds, hazelnuts and oily deep sea fish. Calcium-rich herbs include alfalfa, camomile, oatstraw and skullcap. For women who have cut back on dairy foods because of concerns about weight gain, low-fat alternatives are the ideal substitute. Some women have a deficiency of the lactase enzyme, which means that their bodies are incapable of metabolising dairy products. If you are one of these people you will need to get your calcium from other sources, such as yoghurt, which itself contains the lactase enzyme.

Some food and drinks reduce the availability of calcium to bones. These include large amounts of bran, spinach, broccoli and protein in the diet, more than five cups of coffee a day, and excessive alcohol.

Whatever the source of calcium, taking some of it in the evening will help to minimise bone loss overnight. The traditional warm milky drink before bedtime may have more going for it than merely being an aid to sleep!

People with existing osteoporosis absorb calcium less efficiently than others, and this is often linked with a deficiency of vitamin D, which is produced by the skin in the presence of sunlight. By ensuring regular small amounts of exposure to sun (sometimes a problem for elderly people with mobility problems), or by taking vitamin D in a multivitamin capsule,

Whether or not you are on HRT, you should exercise vigorously, avoid smoking, and eat calcium-rich foods

you can improve calcium absorption. Osteoporosis researchers urge women taking vitamin D supplements not to overdo it, as this can worsen the body's calcium balance.

Various non-hormonal medications are being studied for an effect on bone health, including calcitonin, thiazide, sodium fluoride, anabolic steroids and etidronate. It is too early, as yet, to advocate any of these as an aid to preventing or treating osteoporosis.

Giving up smoking, if they have a cigarette habit, is one of the most helpful things women can do to reduce their risk of developing osteoporosis, according to a US study reported at the Fourth International Symposium on Osteoporosis in 1993. Among a group of nearly 8000 postmenopausal women, those who smoked were nearly three times more likely to sustain a hip fracture than non-smokers when all factors were taken into account. Other research has found that women who do not smoke, or who stop smoking before menopause, cut their risk of a hip fracture by 25 per cent.

Heart and blood vessel health

Regular exercise that stimulates the lungs and blood flow (aerobic exercise) has a beneficial effect on blood clot formation and blood fat levels, lowers blood pressure and reduces the tendency to be overweight. Brisk walking, running, swimming and cycling are all excellent choices. Recent research indicates that muscle-strengthening resistance exercises like weight training also have a favourable effect on blood fat levels.

Reassuringly for those who do not have the urge to run or swim marathons, most of the benefits for heart health occur with moderate exercise programs. You can walk for a total of six hours a week, play golf for five hours or swim for four hours to achieve about the level of activity necessary to provide significant protection against heart disease. Nearly 40 per cent of women around the menopause do not get this amount of exercise, however, if the Melbourne Women's Midlife Health Study is any guide. A further 15 per cent have borderline energy expenditure levels, while just under half have good or very good weekly activity levels.

Smoking endangers heart health, as well as being bad news for bones. If you are a twenty-cigarette-a-day smoker, you will suffer more from atherosclerosis (narrowing and plugging of arteries) than comparable non-smokers. You have double or triple the risk of sustaining a crippling or fatal heart attack than someone of the same age, family history and activity level who does not smoke. Giving up smoking achieves a rapid improvement in heart health. Twelve months after quitting, your risk of sudden death from heart attack is almost half that of persistent smokers and, after five years, this risk is almost identical to that of non-smokers.

Apart from smoking, what you eat and drink are the most important environmental influences on whether or not you will develop heart disease. Healthy eating should not be bland or restrictive, but enjoyable and satisfying. Important features of healthy eating include low levels of fat and sugar and plenty of fresh fruit and vegetables. To reduce the fat content of your meals you should

- remove visible fat from meat and poultry;
- grill, steam, microwave and boil foods rather than frying them;
- use minimal oil and margarine in cooking, sauces and spreads (one to two tablespoons a day);
- eat more fish (but don't fry it!);
- choose low-fat dairy products; and
- limit your intake of 'hidden' fat foods such as processed meats and pastries.

The time of day at which you eat your main meal also seems to be important. A recent study, which compared US and French eating habits, concluded that eating the main meal at lunchtime and snacking only once later may reduce the risk of heart disease. The study is one of a series of investigations into the 'French paradox' – the fact that, despite a diet that is higher in fat than typical diets of other nations, the French have a relatively low rate of death from heart disease. Many Australians get most of their calories at dinner time, watch TV and go to bed. They are sitting on their rear ends or lying horizontally while their main intake of calories is being metabolised. By contrast, the French continue to work for more than five hours after their largest calorie intake, and this is thought to be beneficial for their blood fat levels.

Herbs credited with having a specific effect on the heart and blood vessels include Chinese angelica, ginseng, motherwort and lime blossom. Heart specialists have noted with interest that vitamin E decreases clot formation, which is also an effect of low-dose regular aspirin. Taking both vitamin E and aspirin appears to multiply this effect. Other studies suggest that beta-carotene, a component of fruit and vegetables, also reduces heart attack and stroke risk. Five or more daily servings of fruit and vegetables are required to produce the desired effect.

> ### IN SUMMARY . . .
>
> Many of the suggestions we have made in this chapter – a challenging level of physical activity, not smoking, ample calcium-containing foods and regular pelvic floor exercises, for example – are essential for a vigorous midlife and beyond, whether or not you decide that HRT is right for you.

CHAPTER 7

HRT – why, when, how?

❏ *How do I know if I'm getting near my menopause?*
The most common sign is irregular bleeding – a light period followed by a couple of heavy ones that go on for much longer than usual. You might also notice that you break out in embarrassing hot flushes for no apparent reason. Uncharacteristic moodiness is also quite common, and so are sleeplessness and difficulties with memory or concentration.

❏ *I had an early puberty at the age of eleven. Will this affect the age at which I go through menopause?*
No. The average age of menopause – forty-eight to fifty-three for most Australian women – has changed little over the centuries, while girls now begin their periods at an earlier age than they once did.

❏ *My periods have stopped after several months of irregularity. How long should I wait before having sex without contraception?*

You should use a barrier method of contraception such as condoms or a diaphragm until you have not had a period for a year. You can then throw away your contraceptives.

❏ *I am fifty-five, my periods have stopped, and I don't seem to be noticing menopause. I don't know of any history of heart disease or osteoporosis in my family. Am I a candidate for HRT?*
Probably not. Symptom control and reduction of the long-term risk of fractures or heart disease are the most important reasons for HRT. The view of the Australian Menopause Society is that while most women should consider having HRT for an extended time, 'the most important aspect of menopause management is for the individual woman to be educated and informed about benefits and risks, and to make up her own mind with the help of her informed general practitioner. Benefit clearly outweighs risks for those likely to develop osteoporotic fracture or heart disease but, for those women who have no risk factors for these disorders, the indications to take long-term hormone replacement are not at all clear cut'. Discuss the matter with your own doctor anyway.

❏ *What causes hot flushes?*
The cause is uncertain but the effect is known only too well to millions of women — a rise in skin temperature of 4 to 6 degrees C, a marked increase in heart rate, palpitations, and a reflex opening of the blood vessels to reduce body temperature, giving the skin a flushed appearance. These symptoms tend to clear after a few minutes and may be followed by a feeling of coldness that can lead to shivering.

Hot flushes are likely to peak in the first months to years after the last menstrual bleed, although they also occur in many women who are menstruating regularly. In either case, they provide a good deal of embarrassment and discomfort.

The rate of hot flushes in the non-menopausal female population is about 10 to 20 per cent. For most women the rate of flushes declines rapidly after menopause, although about 10 per cent are still having flushes ten years later, rather longer than most women would like.

We do know that hot flushes parallel an increased output of luteinising hormone (see page 173) produced in a region of the brain that is close to the body's heat centre. There also seems to be a link between flushes and changes to the normal working of blood vessels. One theory links low oestrogen levels with an increase in brain chemicals, leading in turn to a change in the temperature monitoring and regulating part of the brain. This is said to result in the experience of a hot flush, with its associated increase in pulse rate and blood flow to the skin.

Another thing that seems to affect the timing and severity of flushes is anxiety. It is sometimes possible to find connections between anxious situations and the onset of a flush. Stress, the vague state of tension that so much ill health is now put down to, can also increase the tendency to flush. Things that can trigger stress reactions include sleep deprivation, a hot and stuffy environment, thyroid disease and alcohol – common enough factors in anyone's life.

❏ *What causes night sweats, and how are they linked with hot flushes?*
Night sweats are probably hot flushes with the bedclothes on. Flushing and sweating attacks tend to go hand in hand and peak in the years after menopause. The sweating sensation usually takes longer to subside than flushes do.

❏ *Will my hot flushes return with a vengeance if I stop HRT too soon?*

HRT does not seem to affect the duration of hot flushes. If you stop HRT, and you are still in the flushing phase after menopause, your flushes will return. Every woman on HRT for control of hot flushes reaches a point where she wonders if it's time to take a break and see how her body responds. Going off HRT may indicate that the phase of flushes is over or, if not, it will remind you of why you started on HRT in the first place. After a while, of course, the flushes will subside normally – just as they would if you had no HRT.

❏ *I'm told many women give up HRT after a year or two. Why would they do that?*
For a variety of reasons, such as bleeding, a dislike of being on medication for an extended time, and concerns about the long-term possibility of increased risks of breast and endometrial cancers.

❏ *Is there a link between menopause and depression?*
The notion that menopause and depression are linked was a 'fact' commonly stated in medical textbooks well into this century. 'They [menopausal women] are peevish, irritable, morose and depressed', Emil Novak wrote in the classic 1923 text *Menstruation and its Disorders*. 'The various psychoses of the menopause constitute an important group . . . Many [women] have full blown insanity with melancholia, paranoia and maniacal conditions.'

We can laugh now, but such views had a devastating effect on women's lives. Many were placed in psychiatric hospitals for problems that could easily have had more to do with society's weaknesses than theirs. Numerous recent studies have failed to confirm that depressive syndromes increase in middle-aged women. One of the largest studies, conducted by the US National Institute of Mental Health in the 1980s, found that women aged forty-five to sixty-four actually had significantly less depression than men in the same age group.

While fully developed depression is unusual at menopause, 'feeling blue' — or thunderously black — is quite common. It's really hard to separate family stresses and things like financial problems from biological and psychological factors. For some women there seems to be a link between hot flushes, night sweats, insomnia, lethargy, and feeling decidedly depressed. If you are one of these, your cycle of sleeplessness may be broken if you get rid of the flushes with HRT. Even if you are sleeping well, you may find that HRT helps you to dispel uncharacteristically gloomy spells.

❏ *Can HRT help depression?*
It may, particularly if the depressed mood is caused by sleeplessness due to night sweats. However, oestrogen therapy used to treat severe depressive illness has variable results and, when there is severe depressive illness, psychiatric intervention and antidepressant medications are usually needed.

❏ *I am taking oestrogen and progestogen, but I believe the progestogen component is having a depressing effect on my moods and libido. I feel better when I just take the oestrogen. Is this OK?*
Yes, you could consider this as an option, particularly if your withdrawal bleeds are light. However, there is no data to prove that oestrogen without some progestogen is safe for women with a uterus. In the long term you could be increasing your risk of developing cancer of the endometrium by five to ten times, that is, from around one in 1100 to around one in 200. To minimise this possibility, you will need a hysteroscopy and endometrial biopsy every six to twelve months or when any bleeding or spotting occurs.

❏ *Is it necessary to see a specialist about HRT, or is a general practitioner likely to know enough about it?*

In most cases GPs are the best people to advise you on the menopause and HRT, and a specialist referral is usually unnecessary. But not every GP is up to date with these matters because lectures on the menopause have only entered medical school curricula within the last ten years or so.

The growth of menopause clinics (see pages 177–9) may reflect some dissatisfaction among women about the time or information that GPs or gynaecologists provide. These clinics are education-oriented, and most hold regular information sessions for women experiencing menopause or about to do so. Sessions typically cover symptoms, physical changes, HRT, alternative and complementary therapies, diet and exercise, lifestyle changes and relationships. Ideally, women should be able to attend premenopause classes if they want to, just as most attended prenatal classes during pregnancy.

❏ *Instead of taking progestogen each month, is it safe to take it, say, every three to six months so that I don't have so many withdrawal bleeds?*

Researchers are now looking into this possibility. The available evidence suggests that, in some women taking oral oestrogen each day and progestogen for ten to fourteen days every second month, the endometrium is protected sufficiently for this to be a safe and convenient option. Further research is needed to determine which women are best suited for this approach, however. Women who have a very light monthly bleed or no bleed at all could turn out to be suitable. Until the research under way has been completed, it seems likely that most doctors will continue to prescribe some progestogen each month.

❑ *I am taking oestrogen and progestogen, with five days at the end of each cycle when I don't have any hormones. Is this approach widely used?*
There doesn't seem to be any justification for this once-popular approach as menopausal symptoms can return during the hormone 'break'.

❑ *I've had a hysterectomy. Is there any reason why I should take progestogen as part of HRT?*
It was suggested at one stage that progestogen might protect the breast from cancer development, and this remains controversial. At the 8th Congress of the International Menopause Society in Stockholm in 1993 there was considerable discussion of whether oestrogen or progestogen, or both, stimulate breast cell growth. It may be that less stimulation occurs in women on low-dose oestrogen and progestogen throughout each cycle. It was suggested that even women without ovaries should be on this combination. Research is assessing this. Meanwhile women without a uterus usually receive oestrogen alone. This does not seem to increase breast cancer risk in the short term (less than five years).

❑ *I am fed up with hot flushes and night sweats and am considering HRT, but I have fibroids. Should this affect my decision?*
HRT can be prescribed to women with fibroids. However, if fibroids are bulging into the cavity of the uterus heavy bleeding may occur, and this will need to be investigated and may need to be treated before HRT is prescribed.

❑ *My vagina is dry and itchy and sex is often painful. I have started using a vaginal cream that contains oestrogen and wonder if I also need a lubricant?*
You will find that your oestrogen-containing cream improves

lubrication and reduces itchiness within a week or two. Until then, you may want to use a lubricant when having sex.

❏ *Are hysterectomy rates going up?*
After peaking in the late 1970s, rates of hysterectomy appear to have stabilised in Australia, with about 25 per cent of women having the procedure by the age of sixty-five. A NSW study found women aged from thirty-five to forty-nine years were most likely to have it, particularly in their late forties. Most of the operations were for benign disease such as endometriosis or fibroids.

❏ *I have had the lining of my womb removed by laser surgery. Do I need to take progestogen as part of my HRT?*
The technique you describe, endometrial ablation, has been introduced recently into many Australian hospitals. It involves the use of a laser or diathermy (heat) to remove as much of the womb lining – the endometrium – as possible, and is usually considered for women with heavy menstrual bleeding.

Unfortunately there is a misconception that this surgical technique is much the same as a hysterectomy. It isn't. Studies of the uterus after these operations show that some endometrial tissue always remains. This may explain why some patients continue to bleed on and off after an endometrial ablation. It also reinforces the need for future care to protect women from an increased risk of endometrial cancer if they are on HRT after they have had an ablation. A progestogen is required either continuously, in combination with oestrogen, or for ten to fourteen days each month.

❏ *One of my neighbours has had what she calls a total hysterectomy. Does that mean her ovaries as well as her womb have been removed?*

The medical definition of a total hysterectomy is the removal of the uterus and cervix, so your neighbour should still have her ovaries intact. This is the usual type of hysterectomy performed in Australia. If the ovaries are removed along with the uterus and cervix, the procedure is called a hysterectomy plus a bilateral salpingo-oophorectomy.

❑ *Why am I still having heavy monthly bleeds after ten years on HRT?*
A large uterus, and therefore a large surface area of endometrium, is sometimes responsible for heavy bleeds. Another possibility is that fibroids protruding through the endometrium are being stimulated by the hormone therapy to grow and bleed. If you discuss this problem with your doctor, it is likely that he or she will suggest a hysteroscopy (see chapter 2) to check the endometrium. If there is no apparent problem, you may find that your bleeds become lighter with continuous combined HRT (that is, a small dose of oestrogen and progestogen daily).

❑ *I had a couple of clots in my leg fifteen years ago. Should I avoid HRT?*
This depends on whether the clots occurred spontaneously or followed surgery, childbirth or some type of traumatic accident. In either case a thorough assessment of your blood clotting system is called for at the outset.

If the clots appeared 'out of the blue', there is reason for caution with HRT because of the possibility that it may aggravate your clotting disorder and lead to a blocked blood vessel and, at worst, a stroke or heart attack. You may be willing to accept this risk if your menopausal symptoms are particularly severe. If so, the safest HRT option for you is a patch.

If, on the other hand, your clots followed surgery, birth or trauma, it is reasonable to try HRT in patch form after an assessment of your clotting system.

❏ *Adding progestogen to my oestrogen each month gives me a bad headache. What can I do about that?*
Headaches such as you describe are sometimes caused by fluid retention. It may be possible for you to reduce the dose of progestogen you are taking, and this possibility should be raised with your doctor.

❏ *I've had a hysterectomy and I'm taking Premarin pills. Are they likely to raise my blood pressure?*
No, Premarin should not have this effect. If your blood pressure is considered high, it should be treated with a medication for lowering blood pressure and you should continue with your oestrogen.

❏ *Does HRT have any effect on rheumatoid arthritis?*
A number of studies of oestrogens and rheumatoid arthritis have been published, with a mixed set of results. A 1986 study suggested a protective effect, while several more recent studies failed to confirm this. If there is an effect, we don't yet know how long it lasts, whether some methods of delivering HRT to body tissues have a more beneficial effect on this condition than others, or what effect the addition of progestogen may have.

❏ *I've been having HRT to relieve severe hot flushes, and I'm wondering if the dosages are any different from those I need to protect me from osteoporosis or heart disease?*
This depends on the dosage you need to relieve your symptoms, and the individual way your body handles the

hormones. If you are a young woman your symptoms are probably severe, and the dosage you are taking is likely to be ample for protecting your bones and heart. If you are older, your hormone dose may be low and your level of protection may be doubtful. To further complicate the situation, two women of the same age and with similar symptoms may handle the hormones somewhat differently, resulting in a greater level of protection for one or the other.

❏ *Why do women respond to HRT in such a variety of ways?*
This is partly explained by differences in their efficiency at absorbing and metabolising the hormones used in HRT. The slower these processes are, the longer the hormones have to cause adverse effects. Individual differences in responses to oral HRT may also be due to medical conditions – gastric problems, chronic diarrhoea, vomiting or pernicious anaemia, for example – or to interactions with other medications like antibiotics and anti-epileptic drugs.

Your body build also affects the dosage required. Menopausal women who are overweight or have considerable muscular development may need less oestrogen than slim women, because they are producing considerable amounts of oestrogen in fat and muscle tissue, in addition to receiving a small but steady supply of oestrogen from their ovaries.

❏ *I'm thinking of trying HRT. What will my doctor want to know?*
Your doctor will ask whether you have any menopause-related symptoms, such as hot flushes, irregular periods, headaches or dryness of the vagina. It may also be a good idea to discuss other changes in your life at this time. What are your children up to? How about your parents? Are you content with yourself and your place in the family, at work, in the

community? Are all your important relationships in good order? How do you see yourself and your future? That sort of thing.

Your doctor will also check your medical history, including any experience of breast disease such as cysts, breast cancer and so on, and diseases of the reproductive system (cancers of the cervix, uterus or ovaries, fibroids, endometriosis, premenstrual syndrome and so on). He or she will also want to know whether you have had any abnormal blood clotting or high blood pressure, including elevated blood pressure during pregnancy (pre-eclampsia).

Your menstrual history is also of interest, and so are any experiences of anorexia, menstrual periods disappearing for longer than six months, and long-term use of steroids – for example, for the treatment of asthma or thyroid disease.

❏ *What are the advantages of the oestrogen patch over oral oestrogen?*
The patch is worth trying if you don't tolerate oral oestrogen well (side effects like nausea, abdominal pain or headaches will tell you that). You're much less likely to have these side effects with the patch because it cuts down the number of times the oestrogen passes through your liver. This means that the liver is not stimulated so much to produce proteins that may interfere with normal blood pressure and your fluid control systems.

The patch may also be more convenient than taking oestrogen tablets each day, because it is applied twice a week.

All the same, oral oestrogen is the way most doctors prefer to start patients who need oestrogen therapy. The main reason is that there is considerable research demonstrating the effectiveness of oestrogen pills in managing menopausal symptoms and protecting the bones, heart and blood vessels.

Regrettably, research on HRT patch formulations has not been going on for long. Recent studies indicate that the patch protects against osteoporosis if you use it for longer than six months, but so far there is very little long-term data regarding its impact on heart and blood vessel disease.

❏ *I am nearly sixty and am thinking of starting on HRT. Will I need smaller or larger hormone doses than I would have needed ten years ago when I went through menopause?*
It's likely that your hormone requirements and tolerance will both be somewhat lower than they were ten years ago. This is not the case for women who have been having HRT continuously since menopause: their needs and tolerance will not change much in ten years.

Having said that, your dose will depend on why you are thinking of starting HRT. If it's for symptom control, you will need lower doses than if the main reason is to prevent or control osteoporosis or heart and blood vessel disease.

❏ *Will HRT make me look younger, by removing facial wrinkles for example?*
HRT will not remove wrinkles, but over a period of some months it may improve the texture and thickness of skin by increasing the collagen in it so that the skin looks fuller. An estimated 15 to 30 per cent of collagen is lost from the skin in the first five years after menopause. The best way to prevent wrinkles forming is to avoid excessive sun exposure, wear a hat, and use sunblocks and moisturisers.

❏ *If I forgot to take my oestrogen tablets for a week, would I notice any difference?*
Any symptoms you had before starting on HRT would probably return within a matter of days.

❏ *Do we know enough about the long-term effects of HRT to be sure it's safe and will live up to the claims made for it?*
One area of concern is a possible increased risk of breast cancer in women on HRT for more than ten years. This is an issue that many research teams are investigating (it is discussed in detail in chapter 4).

Another area of uncertainty is the effect on heart disease risk of including progestogens in HRT formats. It seems that while progestogens protect the endometrium, they may also reduce the protective effects of oestrogen on blood fats when used in large doses. The 19-nortestosterone progestogens (see page 176) seem to have a more adverse effect than the more commonly prescribed Provera in this regard.

It is also unclear what effects long-term use of progestogens (high or low dose) have on women. Studies are under way in many medical and research centres worldwide, including several in Australia, but we won't know the answer to this question until the end of this decade.

❏ *I've decided to try HRT after discussing my situation with my doctor. Is there any particular time after menopause when it's best to start?*
If you are having menopausal symptoms that interfere with your quality of life, you can start on HRT at any time. If the main reason for HRT is your worry about a high risk of osteoporosis or heart disease in the future, it's best to start on it within about twelve months of your menopause. It's also acceptable to begin at any time *after* the menopausal years. For example, a woman in her late sixties whose bone density is found to be critically low can start HRT to prevent any further loss of calcium from her bones.

❏ *My periods are getting less regular and I'm wondering whether there's any sense in starting HRT before they finally stop. Could I avoid menopausal symptoms by doing this, for example?*
This is not recommended, because many women don't develop any significant menopausal symptoms and are not at risk of heart disease or osteoporosis, the other main reason for having HRT. Another reason why we don't normally offer HRT before menopause is that women could end up with persistently high levels of oestrogen, and we don't know the effects of this yet.

❏ *How long should I stay on HRT?*
That depends on why you are having it. If it's to control symptoms, you'll probably need HRT for between two and ten years, depending on how long the symptoms last. If it's for protection of your bones, heart and blood vessels, your doctor will probably recommend that you stay on HRT until your late sixties or early seventies, or for the rest of your life.

❏ *When should I stop HRT for symptom control?*
When you feel comfortable about it. If you don't want to go on any longer because it gives you side effects, or you feel well and are reluctant to continue taking pills, using patches or whatever, it's a good idea to see how you get on without them. If you do stop HRT, the dose of hormones should be gradually reduced.

❏ *Should I take my HRT pills at the same time each day?*
Yes. This seems to give better control of symptoms and reduces the likelihood of spotting.

❏ *Will I need to change the type of HRT I'm on, or the dosage, as time goes by, even though it seems to suit me well?*

No. Once a hormone format is found that suits a particular woman's needs, she is usually advised to stay with that format unless an alternative is developed that is likely to suit her better. Your dosage will probably also remain unchanged unless you have unwanted side effects at some stage.

❏ *Can I use a hormone-based vaginal cream if I'm already using an oestrogen patch?*
A vaginal cream used twice a week together with a patch may be called for if vaginal dryness is particularly troublesome and the oestrogen patch on its own does not do the trick.

❏ *Do I need to remove my HRT patch when I shower or swim?*
Patches are designed to withstand the sorts of activities you describe, but if you find there is a problem, remove it from your skin and replace it on its original backing while you shower or swim. When you've dried off, put it back on again.

❏ *Is there any evidence that HRT reduces the risk of bowel cancer?*
Several studies suggest that oestrogen confers substantial protection against bowel cancer, while at least one other well-designed study has not reproduced this finding. Various groups of researchers are currently attempting to come up with a conclusive answer to this important question.

❏ *I understand that endometriosis becomes less of a problem after menopause without any treatment. Does HRT make a difference?*
Endometriosis present at the time of menopause usually disappears after it. In exceptional cases, adhesions caused by endometriosis may continue to cause problems. If oestrogen is given from the time of menopause, there is a theoretical risk of stimulating the endometriosis, but in practice this rarely

occurs. Taking oestrogen and progestogen together every day is likely to be less stimulatory than taking cyclical progestogen (for ten to fourteen days of each cycle).

❏ *I have developed patches of discoloured skin since using oestrogen. Is this normal? Will it go away when I come off hormone therapy?*
Many women on oestrogen (in contraceptive pill or HRT form) are dismayed to find that patches of coloured pigment appear on their skin after they have spent time in the sun. This is called chloasma, and is caused by deposits of melanin in the skin. In a small proportion of women, oestrogen seems to stimulate chloasma development. The effect will usually fade when you stop taking oestrogen, but this depends on how much exposure you have to the sun. Always use a sunblock: your doctor or pharmacist may suggest an anti-chloasma type.

❏ *Are lumpy breasts a reason not to take oestrogen?*
No . . . but whether you use oestrogen or not, it is important to examine your breasts regularly, have your doctor check them over too (at least annually), have regular mammograms and avoid smoking.

❏ *I have had breast cancer. Is there any form of therapy, including HRT, that might help to control the severe flushes I am having?*
HRT is sometimes considered for women who've had breast cancer, particularly if quality of life is the priority and nothing else works to reduce flushes. In these cases, Provera or low doses of natural oestrogens (and daily progestogen if you have a uterus) are likely to be chosen. If your breast surgeon and oncologist feel you should not use HRT, you might like to try regular exercise, evening primrose oil or pressed linseed oil,

vitamin E, relaxation and meditation to control your flushes. The prescription medication clonidine may also be helpful.

❏ *Since starting on Estigyn eleven years ago I have developed benign cysts in one breast. Is it possible that HRT caused this problem? Should I change my therapy or come off HRT altogether?*
There is no evidence that oestrogen, even the synthetic form of oestrogen you are on, causes breast cysts. However, oestrogen may stimulate the growth of existing breast abnormalities like cysts or fibroadenomas, causing them to become larger and more obvious. You should certainly consider changing the type of oestrogen you use. Estigyn is a powerful synthetic oestrogen and, as we explained in chapter 2, it is more likely to produce side effects than a natural oestrogen formulation. There is no justification for you to come off HRT in the circumstances you describe.

❏ *The reason I am taking oestrogen is to make sure that my bone strength is maintained. How can I be certain that the dosage of oestrogen is high enough?*
The only reliable way is to have two bone density scans twelve to eighteen months apart. This will indicate whether your bone density has been maintained or has deteriorated while you have been on HRT. If the density has fallen, your dose of oestrogen should be increased if there are no medical reasons against this.

❏ *Should all women contemplating HRT have a bone density scan?*
No, it is unrealistic for every woman contemplating HRT to ask for a bone density scan as the procedure is offered by only a small number of centres and the cost to women varies from

about $30 to over $100. The federal government is considering introducing a Medicare rebate for the procedure. What's more important is that it's not necessary for every woman.

Those for whom bone density scans are appropriate have one or more of the following characteristics:
- a family history of osteoporosis
- an experience of breaking a bone around the time of menopause with very little force applied
- strong risk factors for osteoporosis, such as a history of absent periods for six or more months, heavy smoking, excessive alcohol or caffeine consumption, prolonged immobilisation and a poor diet
- difficulty deciding whether or not to remain on HRT now that symptom control is no longer the purpose for it

There may also be some women without symptoms who are contemplating HRT, and the bone density measurement will help them make their decision.

❏ *Will Medicare cover all my menopausal tests and treatments?*
Medicare covers all investigations except bone density scans, and this may change in the near future.

❏ *Can premenopausal women increase their bone strength? The reason I ask is that my bone density is low, possibly due to a time many years ago when I was anorexic and didn't have periods for over a year.*
You are right in thinking that your low bone density probably relates to the time when you were anorexic, which is likely to have had an adverse effect on your peak bone mass. With the current state of knowledge about osteoporosis, the most helpful things to do at this stage are to make sure your diet is nutritious and well balanced, with plenty of calcium-containing foods (see chapter 6), to avoid smoking, to exer-

cise regularly, and to get regular sun exposure, which will help your body make vitamin D (essential for calcium absorption).

❑ *If peak bone density occurs between twenty and thirty years in women, what should I do to ensure that the bones of my daughters are as strong as possible?*
You should be educating your daughters now about the need to eat nutritious foods rich in calcium. The recommended daily calcium intake for girls of eight to eleven is 900 mg (boys need 800 mg), which is equivalent to three or four daily serves of calcium-rich food (one serve can be 250 mL milk, 200 g yoghurt or 35 g cheese). Girls aged twelve to fifteen years should have around 1000 mg daily (boys 1200 mg), which is four to five serves of calcium-rich food. For women aged sixteen to fifty, three serves daily or 800 mg of calcium-rich food suffice (the same for men of all ages), and from fifty onwards women should increase their intake of calcium-rich foods to four or five serves (1000–1500 mg).

It is also important to remember that the growth patterns of boys and girls vary, with girls starting their spurt at around the age of eleven and boys later, at around thirteen. So an eleven-year-old girl will probably be eating more than her twelve-year-old brother. It's important to realise this, otherwise parents may be critical of a daughter's appetite.

Girls also tend to be excessively concerned about the amount of body fat they acquire during adolescence. They need reassurance that fat on breasts, legs and hips is normal. Otherwise they may turn to fad diets or excessive exercise and quickly become deficient in energy, protein, calcium and iron. In extreme cases this may lead to anorexia nervosa. Regular moderate exercise will improve appearance, even if it means gaining weight in terms of muscle.

❏ *I have reduced my intake of dairy products because there's heart disease in my family, and I'm concerned about the effect this may have on my bones. What alternative sources of calcium can you suggest?*
Calcium-rich non-dairy foods include tinned fish with bones, oysters, nuts and seeds. You should eat them with your evening meal: other foods will help the process of calcium absorption. Vitamin D, obtained from an action of sunlight on the skin, also helps calcium absorption, while too much dietary fibre, spinach or broccoli interferes with it. Calcium is needed consistently on a daily basis, so make sure that whatever you do to keep up your supplies takes account of this.

Of course you could confine your eating of dairy foods to non-fat forms, and still get plenty of calcium from them without increasing the risk of heart disease.

❏ *When should prevention of osteoporosis start?*
Osteoporosis prevention should start in childhood, and there are a number of things that can be done to build stronger bones. These include encouraging children (boys as well as girls) to eat foods rich in calcium such as milk, cheese, yoghurt and fish with bones, and to take regular exercise. Sadly, many older women now suffering from osteoporosis were brought up at a time when there was little emphasis on a well-balanced diet and regular weight-bearing exercise. Many took as gospel the misguided words of the Duchess of Windsor, 'You can never be too thin or too rich'.

More than 50 per cent of Australian women (and 30 per cent of Australian men) consume less than the recommended dietary intake of calcium. For teenagers it's no better, with nearly a third of fifteen-year-old girls getting less than half the calcium they need, according to a national dietary survey of Australian schoolchildren aged from ten to fifteen years.

❑ *Does HRT have a lasting effect on bone strength, or will it only maintain the strength of my bones while I'm on it?*
Adequate dosages of HRT hormones maintain bone density, but only while you are taking them. Once you stop HRT, you'll lose bone density at the rate that would have occurred if you had never started on it. HRT therefore only postpones bone loss to a later age.

❑ *Is HRT any help in stopping established osteoporosis from getting worse?*
Yes, it can stabilise bone density, even if you start it at the age of eighty or so.

❑ *Does having a hysterectomy make any difference to heart disease risk?*
There is little doubt that hysterectomy increases the risk of cardiovascular disease. This may be true not only for women who have their ovaries removed but also for those in whom the ovaries are preserved. Given the evidence about a benefit to the heart from use of oestrogen, it is particularly important that these women have access to it.

❑ *How can I work out whether or not I am especially likely to get heart disease or osteoporosis, or both?*
There are two sorts of risk to consider: your inherited risk, determined by your genetic make-up, and your acquired risk, influenced by your lifestyle.

First, if you don't already know, you should try to find out whether any of your close relatives – parents, grandparents, brothers, sisters, uncles, aunts – have died prematurely of heart or blood vessel disease or have broken any bones at or after middle age. If so, you may be at increased risk of heart disease or osteoporosis. Slight body build and northern European background also increase your chances of osteoporosis.

Second, you should consider lifestyle factors that influence the development of these problems. Smoking is bad news because it reduces the density of bones as well as damaging the heart and blood vessels. How much you smoke or smoked and for how long will affect your risk.

Nutritional factors, such as a diet rich in animal fat, are associated with an increased risk of heart and blood vessel disease. And so is a hysterectomy, whether or not you had your ovaries removed. A low calcium intake during the teenage and early adult years, a personal experience of anorexia nervosa, the absence of menstrual periods for longer than six months during the teen years or adulthood, and heavy use of alcohol or caffeine are all linked with a greater likelihood of osteoporosis and fractures. Being immobilised for long periods, or simply having a lifestyle with limited exercise also increases this risk.

While family history and lifestyle are important in assessing your risk of osteoporosis, there is also a bone density scan available if your fracture risk seems high. This can be carried out in many x-ray departments, or at specialised menopause centres such as those listed on pages 177–9.

Likewise, as regards your risk of heart disease, you should consider a check of your blood fats, including cholesterol, to add to the information you already have about your family history and lifestyle risk factors. A difficulty here is that most of the research on the link between blood fat levels and heart disease has been conducted on men, and recent findings suggest that cholesterol levels considered unacceptably high in men may not represent as serious a danger for women.

Another difficulty with heart disease risk analysis is that only about half the people with risk factors like high blood pressure and high cholesterol actually develop heart disease.

Work is under way to find accurate methods of predicting who will develop heart disease and who won't. One promising method involves monitoring the length of time people take to eliminate fats from the bloodstream: this clearance time seems to be related to heart disease risk.

If you are not experiencing any menopausal symptoms, or very few symptoms, but you have a high risk of fractures or heart and blood vessel disease, there are a number of things you need to weigh up, bearing in mind your own values and needs. Think, on the one hand, of the protection HRT offers against bone thinning or heart disease and, on the other, of the commitment needed to stay for many years on a therapy that will produce no immediate benefits and may give you an increased breast cancer risk if used long-term; you may also have to take into account nuisance withdrawal bleeds, as well as side effects including nausea and breakthrough bleeding.

❏ *Men's risk of heart disease is much greater than women's, so why don't they use some form of hormone therapy to reduce the risk?*
Trials of oestrogen therapy have been conducted on men, but the doses used were inappropriately high. This caused harm to some participants and the enthusiasm for such trials seems to have waned.

Oestrogen used to treat prostate cancer increases the risk of cardiovascular disease in men, though the doses are very high and the types of oestrogen used are not necessarily those likely to be beneficial to healthy men. It can also cause growth of breasts and suppression of sex drive and potency.

❏ *How can I know if I'm at risk of breast cancer?*
Breast cancer is more likely if you have a family history of the disease (for example, a mother or sisters who have suffered

from it). If you have had a previous breast cancer yourself, you are also more likely than average to have cancer in the other breast. Your risk also tends to be greater if you are white, urban, educated or childless; if you started having periods earlier than usual or your menopause occurred at an above-average age; or if you have ever had any abnormal cells in a breast biopsy.

❑ *I took oestrogen for five years during the 1980s to help me cope with menopausal symptoms. Now I read that I should have been taking progestogen as well to protect my uterus from cancer. Can I do anything about it now?*
Go and see your doctor, who may prescribe a progestogen like Provera for ten to twelve days to check whether any vaginal bleeding follows. If it does, it means that your uterus still has some endometrium – the old lining – and an investigation such as diagnostic hysteroscopy and biopsy will need to be done (see chapter 2). If there's no bleeding, there is not likely to be a problem. An oestrogen measurement and an ultrasound to check the thickness of your endometrium may also be in order.

❑ *How soon after I start on HRT can I expect my symptoms to improve?*
Most women prescribed an appropriate hormone dose see a response within a week of starting. If the dose prescribed is too low, however, improvements may take longer.

❑ *How is HRT likely to improve in the next few years?*
The most likely changes include the following:
- new combinations of oestrogens and progestogens that do not promote bleeding, minimise other unwanted effects, yet benefit bone, heart and blood vessels;

- packs that include oestrogen patches and progestogen patches or tablets in new delivery systems that reduce side effects and are based on long-term studies of safety and cancer risk; and
- new options for progestogen-sensitive patients.

❏ *Convince me that HRT is not a cynical exercise in medicalisation, by pharmaceutical and medical interests, of a perfectly normal part of a woman's life.*

For many women HRT is their salvation from symptoms that put barriers in the way of living a normal life. Women should not be denied access to this therapy, nor should they feel guilty about using it. But the idea that all women should have HRT is simplistic. Each woman needs to be assessed individually. At the same time she should be given sound information about the non-medical alternatives to HRT.

Menopause is a natural part of life, but that doesn't stop it being a major impediment to quality living for a proportion of women, particularly those who have had an early menopause, surgical or natural .

It's true that HRT is big business for the pharmaceutical companies, and this means that doctors have to be very careful to present the facts to women in a clear and unbiased way. Cynics might say that doctors and pharmaceutical companies are more interested in their bank balances than in treating debilitating symptoms or protecting women from future bone, heart and blood vessel problems. But separating self-interest from the patient's interests is, of course, an important part of all medical practice. It's up to women to make sure they get clear and accurate information so that they can make an informed choice about how to manage their own lives. If this information is not forthcoming from your doctor, perhaps it is time to look elsewhere.

❏ *How can I be sure that the mistakes made with previous formats of HRT are not now being repeated for a new generation of women?*
It is unfortunately all too true that the oestrogen replacement therapy widely prescribed in Australia, the US and UK until the late 1970s caused a significant number of cases of endometrial cancer. This form of cancer may develop when oestrogen is used alone without progestogen by women who have an intact uterus.

Medical practitioners know considerably more today than they did then about the role of various reproductive hormones and their relationship with cancer and other diseases. While more is known, we are still on a learning curve with HRT. Here's just one example. Recent research indicates that the actions of classic hormones like oestrogen and progesterone do not fully explain the way the reproductive system works. A large number of other hormones such as inhibin (see page 174) can apparently fine-tune the way the body responds to the classic hormones. It is only within the past decade that some of these local hormones have been identified, and there may be others as yet undiscovered.

❏ *I have read a doctor's comment that an important reason for prescribing HRT is to help reduce the amount of money spent on the care of elderly women. Do you agree?*
There is no doubt that care of elderly women is a significant part of health care spending. But what is often neglected in these financial analyses is the enormous amounts of money these same women save the health care system by looking after sick and dying husbands or other family members at home, often for many years.

Such comments also imply that long-term HRT will necessarily result in a fitter, healthier group of older women. We don't yet have the evidence to say this with certainty. It may be that widespread use of HRT will result in women living longer and with fewer fractures and heart attacks. However, nothing is more certain than that we must all die, and if the cause of death is not heart disease or complications from fractures, it could well be a disease that might cost the community even more, such as dementia or cancer.

❏ *Is there anything to suggest that society's attitudes to women at midlife are changing?*
Attitudes to physical beauty still seem harsher for women in their middle years than for men of the same age. We are so geared to youth, and youth is so tied up with femininity and sexuality, that once you reach menopause you may be viewed as 'past it'.

The environmentalist and anti-nuclear campaigner Dr Helen Caldicott, whose marriage of twenty-six years broke up on the eve of her fiftieth birthday, says blinkered attitudes do not help. 'In the eyes of some men, older women . . . have lost almost all value when they reach menopause because their hormones are no longer at the level they were before.' Dr Caldicott has achieved a new beginning and a sense of liberation and independence since moving out of the family home, to settle first on the north-east coast of New South Wales and then in Gippsland, Victoria. 'Doing it released me and made me understand the strength I had.'

Women actors complain that few challenging roles are available once they reach about forty-five. While men such as Sean Connery, Sam Neill and Robert Redford still play romantic leads into and beyond their fifties, women are rarely seen in such parts. Genevieve Picot, who played the role of the obsessive Celia in *Proof* and is deputy federal president of the Actors Equity section of the Media, Entertainment & Arts

Alliance, says she is frustrated about being considered 'old' in the industry. 'The irony and the disappointment for me is that as a performer I'm feeling much more confident and my skills are so much better than they were ten or fifteen years ago, yet I just don't have the opportunity to use them very much.'

There are signs of change, however, the most obvious place being on television, where presenters and commentators are increasingly likely to include women over forty who do not necessarily look like stunners.

The highly regarded SBS newsreader Mary Kostakidis believes women themselves must make the first move. She refuses to dye her greying hair because she sees no point in camouflaging the maturity and complexity that come with midlife and beyond. 'As a younger woman I was often attracted to older men because of these sorts of qualities. And now that I've arrived there myself, I'm not about to cover up the fact.'

She says that women presenters on Australian television are still largely ornamental. 'It's boring. We are an ageing population, and decision-makers who cannot accept this and act accordingly are behind the times. In many cultures older women assume positions of great status and respect. Australian women also have pride in their years. The time must come when they are no longer discarded for no other reason than their age. If not – if our institutions don't reflect our values – our democracy is a farce.'

Women throughout Australia are, like Mary, Helen and Genevieve, asking questions, getting information, and deciding what is important for them at midlife and beyond.

CHAPTER 8

Your choice

*H*AVE YOU EVER been on your way to an appointment when the car radio has blared out details of a traffic snarl on your intended route? A series of questions probably flashed through your mind. How serious is the hold-up? How long will it take to clear? Can I bypass the trouble spot? What are the alternative routes? How likely are they to be congested? What detours must I make to get to another route? Life is full of choices made under conditions of uncertainty.

Decisions about medical treatment such as HRT demand a more careful approach than choosing the route to an appointment, but psychologists tell us that the decision-making process has much in common with that described above. You form a set of expectations about the likelihood of particular outcomes, bearing in mind uncertainties about the information available. You place a particular weight on one or other of those outcomes. You take into consideration other factors that are important to you, for example the inconvenience of this approach or that, the costs involved, the effort of remembering when to do what, the experiences of your friends and others whose judgement you trust.

When Dale Spender, whom we first met in chapter 1, was deciding whether or not to try HRT in her early forties, some of the considerations she took into account included the following:

- her experience of menopause, which was of drenching sweats and hot flushes that were messing up her life; and
- her expectations of HRT, which included both positive features — like relief from her symptoms — and negative possibilities such as an increased risk of breast cancer.

'Any responsible human being knows that taking drugs on a daily basis is not without risk,' she told a magazine in 1991. 'There is not a drug on the market that has not been hailed as a wonder drug and then found wanting some years later.' Dale's decision to try HRT was not the end of the story. Although the flushes and sweats eased and her life returned to 'something like a normal existence', her breasts were unbearably sore. At her doctor's suggestion she bought a cabbage, went home, tore off a few leaves and wrapped them around her breasts. 'The smell! I can't tell you. But it was no good. Nothing is.'

All in all she found the sweats more debilitating than the sore breasts, and she planned to stay on HRT until the age of fifty-two, when she would reassess the situation. Her experi-

Decisions about HRT have the potential to affect the daily lives of women, and perhaps also their future health and wellbeing

ence of making decisions about HRT in a situation where some things are known and others are uncertain, and where some of the evidence is conflicting, is common to many women at and after menopause.

The balance sheet

In deciding about HRT, the following points should be taken into account.

- HRT is effective in relieving hot flushes and night sweats, vaginal dryness and urinary symptoms.
- It is particularly helpful to women who have had a premature menopause (either natural or medically induced). They are likely to benefit most from HRT both because they tend to suffer more extreme symptoms of menopause and are at increased risk of osteoporosis and diseases of the heart and blood vessels, and because in many cases they no longer have a uterus and so the hormone therapy is simpler.
- Oestrogen used on its own seems to confer a worthwhile degree of protection against heart and blood vessel disease. This benefit is heightened for women who have had a hysterectomy and in whom there is no added risk of endometrial cancer.
- The decision about which HRT preparation is suitable for the larger number of women who have not had a hysterectomy depends on the balance between several potential benefits and hazards. On both scores, there are gaps in information that research will start to fill during the remainder of this decade.
- In deciding whether to undertake HRT for prolonged periods in the absence of worrisome symptoms, women should take account of both the anticipated benefits and the possible risks. On the benefit side, oestrogen use post-

pones bone thinning and reduces the likelihood of heart disease. When it is combined with a progestogen, there are still significant benefits for bones, but progestogen appears to negate some of the protective effect that oestrogen has on the cardiovascular system.

On the risk side, the biggest concerns lie with cancers of the breast and endometrium. Breast cancer is the most common cancer of the reproductive organs and the one most feared by women, so consideration of the link between oestrogen and breast cancer is tremendously important in helping

Women will make decisions based on their family history of disease, their own life experiences and education, and the advice of others they trust

women to decide about HRT. Statistical studies indicate that the number of women whose lives will be saved by HRT, through a reduction in serious bone breaks and heart attacks, is much greater than the number who will die through cancer. However if, for a particular woman, the avoidance of an increased cancer risk is more important than the numerically greater benefit in terms of osteoporosis or cardiovascular disease, this is clearly the basis on which her treatment should be decided.

- For many women, drawbacks to combined oestrogen and progestogen include withdrawal bleeding, breakthrough bleeding and PMS-like side effects.
- For women who use oestrogen on its own and who still have a uterus, an important consideration is the need for regular and extended monitoring of their gynaecological health.

Final words

Menopause is a powerful marker of age, and the end of menstrual periods confronts women with their own ageing more dramatically than any biological process experienced by men. This is at once a boon and a problem. It may be regarded as a boon because it can trigger a stocktaking by women that allows them to recognise the importance of taking on new challenges. A major problem is that society's attitudes to women at and after menopause, and women's own attitudes and experience of this stage of life, can trigger feelings of anxiety for the future, diminished self-confidence and grief.

In talking to women generally, and more specifically to those seeking medical advice, we have clearly seen that the significance of menopause extends beyond an end to the possibility of having children. From childhood and adolescence onwards, we learn to attach great significance to our sex hormones, developing an uncanny ability to tune into them. We can often 'tell' when our periods are approaching, when we are ovulating, when we have become pregnant.

The notion that our ovaries, a major source of our sex hormones, effectively 'die' at menopause, leaving us in a state of hormonal deficiency, is incorrect, except in women whose ovaries are removed or irreparably impaired. In general, sex hormone output after menopause settles to a lower but still quite measurable level. It makes sense that there should be some change, for we are no longer ovulating, menstruating or conceiving.

Hormone replacement therapy can seem like a lifeline both for women who do not have functioning ovaries and for other women. It promises relief from severe symptoms, it can improve our coping abilities, and can perhaps prevent some of the future health problems we worry about. As with most medications, however, there are uncertainties, and unwanted effects sometimes.

The Australian Menopause Society recommends that most women should consider HRT, not for a year or two, but for a minimum of five to fifteen years and probably for longer. Other authorities, like the Key Centre for Women's Health in Society at the University of Melbourne, are more cautious. As its director, Professor Lorraine Dennerstein, explained to a packed lecture theatre of middle-aged and older women at the University of Melbourne in 1992, more information is needed about the long-term effects of HRT formulations, and about the dosages now being used. 'HRT does relieve debilitating symptoms, but a lot of work needs to be done on dosage and there is much that women can do to minimise symptoms themselves.'

In this atmosphere of uncertainty, women are faced with decisions about whether or not to use HRT, decisions that have the potential to affect their daily lives and perhaps also their future health and wellbeing. This book aims to peel back the layers of half-truth and confusion that surround HRT, so that women retain in their own hands the power to decide and a belief in their own ability to do so.

APPENDIX

Sex hormone levels after menopause

There is considerable variability in the sex hormone levels of postmenopausal women. In general, postmenopausal women whose ovaries are intact produce levels of ovarian hormones (except for oestradiol) comparable with those they produced in the early part of their menstrual cycle prior to menopause. The main difference between this group and those women who have had a surgical menopause is that the second group produce smaller amounts of the hormones known as androgens.

Oestrogen hormones

The change in the oestrogen hormone profile is a matter of altered balance between the various types of oestrogen produced.

OESTRONE This is the most constant form of oestrogen circulating in the bloodstream from childhood onwards. In postmenopausal women (with or without ovaries), its level is about the same as in the early part of the menstrual cycle before menopause. (Much higher levels occur at mid-cycle and in the late part of the cycle.) It is mainly produced from androgens (described later) in muscle and fat tissue. This is why body fat is a major factor in determining oestrogen levels in postmenopausal women. The ovaries (if present) produce some oestrone too.

OESTRADIOL Oestradiol is the most powerful of the oestrogen hormones and it has the greatest influence on the function of the heart and blood vessels, bone growth, brain metabolism, reproduction and menstruation. A postmenopausal woman (with ovaries) has about half the level she had in the early part of her menstrual cycle, which is about one-tenth of the average level for the whole menstrual cycle. Oestradiol levels of women without ovaries are somewhat lower.

Oestradiol is mainly converted from oestrone in fat and muscle tissue throughout the body, and from androgens in the adrenal glands – two small organs above the kidneys. Hot flushes and night sweats typically correspond with low levels of oestradiol.

OESTRIOL A third type of oestrogen produced in large amounts by the placenta during pregnancy is called oestriol. It is a weak form of oestrogen and is converted from oestrone. It is present in measurable amounts both before and after menopause in women with and without ovaries.

Follicle Stimulating Hormone and Luteinising Hormone

The output of these hormones is much greater after menopause than beforehand.

FOLLICLE STIMULATING HORMONE (FSH) This acts on the ovary and triggers the ripening of follicles that contain eggs, thus setting the stage for ovulation during the fertile years. FSH is not one substance but a group of more than twenty similar substances produced by the pituitary gland of the brain. Scientists are only just starting to study the multiple forms of FSH and to assess their roles at different stages of life. In the fertile years, high levels of oestradiol and inhibin (described later) suppress the brain's output of FSH. When the output of oestradiol and inhibin declines after menopause, there is less suppression of FSH production and its level in the bloodstream increases to ten or fifteen times that seen in the early part of the premenopausal menstrual cycle. The rise is gradual at first, then reaches a peak at which it stays for three to five years after menopause. It returns to the premenopausal range twenty or so years later.

LUTEINISING HORMONE (LH) Best known as the hormone with final responsibility for release of the ripened egg at ovulation, it also stimulates the ovaries to produce androgens and plays a part in their conversion to oestradiol. Like FSH, LH is produced by the brain and is not just a single substance (there are more than forty slightly different forms). Before menopause, high levels of oestradiol suppress the brain's output of LH. When oestradiol levels drop after menopause, LH levels rise. Large shifts in LH levels are associated with hot flushes. Postmenopausal LH levels peak about two years after menopause, and then gradually return to the premenopausal range during the following twenty years. The peak postmenopausal level is still less than the mid-cycle peak occurring before menopause.

Progesterone

With the approach of menopause and less frequent ovulation, production of progesterone by the ovaries dwindles. However, the level of progesterone after menopause is similar to that of the early part of the menstrual cycle in the fertile years. This progesterone is produced by the adrenal glands.

Androgens

There are three kinds of androgen, and the balance changes after menopause. Overall, the level of androgens produced at that stage is lower than beforehand, with a more marked reduction in women who have had a surgical menopause.

Because testosterone is the most dominant androgen, and because its level after menopause is still relatively high, it plays a rather more dominant role in the sex hormone system after the menopause than beforehand.

ANDROSTENEDIONE This is the most constant androgen before and after menopause and is the main source of postmenopausal oestrogen. The level of androstenedione after menopause is about half that present during the early part of the menstrual cycle. It is a little lower in women who have had a surgical menopause. The ovaries produce androstenedione after menopause in response to high levels of LH. The adrenal glands also produce it both before and after menopause.

TESTOSTERONE The most powerful of the androgen hormones, testosterone influences hair growth, voice and libido in women. The level of testosterone after menopause tends to be a little less than it was during the early part of the menstrual cycle. The level after surgical menopause is about half that after natural menopause. The testosterone of postmenopausal women is produced by both the ovaries and the adrenal glands.

DEHYDRO EPIANDROSTERONE (DHA) This is produced by the adrenal glands before and after menopause, and its output falls to about a third through the menopause transition.

Inhibin

Inhibin is a recently discovered ovarian hormone with two major roles. It signals information to the brain about the state of egg production in the ovaries, and helps to regulate this process by controlling the level of FSH. After the menopause its level drops, which helps to explain why the level of FSH rises.

Hormones commonly used in HRT, with trade names and typical dosage range

In general, smaller dosages are appropriate for older women.

Oestrogens

NATURAL OESTROGENS	TYPICAL DOSAGE RANGE
oestradiol valerate (Progynova)	1–4 mg daily
conjugated equine oestrogen (Premarin)	0.3–2.5 mg daily
piperazine oestrone sulphate (Ogen)	0.625–2.5 mg daily
micronised oestradiol (a component of Trisequens or Trisequens Forte)	1–4 mg daily, depending on stage of cycle
transdermal oestradiol (Estraderm patch)	25, 50 and 100 mcg absorbed daily and changed twice weekly
subcutaneous oestradiol (Oestradiol implant)	20–100 mg inserted at intervals between every 3 months and every 12 months

SYNTHETIC OESTROGEN	
ethinyl oestradiol (Estigyn)	0.01–0.03 mg daily

Progestogens

These may be taken every day or for 10 to 14 days a cycle.

C-21 DERIVATIVES

medroxyprogesterone acetate (Provera)	*2.5–20 mg daily*
dydrogesterone (Duphaston)	*10–20 mg daily*

19-NORTESTOSTERONE DERIVATIVES

levonorgestrel (Microlut, Microval)	*0.03–0.09 mg daily*
norethisterone (Primolut, Micronor or Noriday)	*0.35–5 mg daily*
norethisterone acetate (Trisequens or Trisequens Forte)	*1 mg on 10 days of cycle*

THIRD-GENERATION OR TERTIARY PROGESTOGENS

desogestrel (a component of the oral contraceptive Marvelon)	*not yet available in Australia for HRT*

ANTI-ANDROGENS

cyproterone acetate (Androcur)	*1–5 mg daily*

Substances with the function of oestrogen or progestogen or both

OD14 or tibolone (Livial)	*not yet available in Australia*

If vaginal creams are prescribed, the dosages will be low to prevent a possible stimulatory effect on the endometrium. The low-dose therapy usually consists of conjugated equine oestrogen (Premarin) cream, 1–2 g, two to three times a week; or Ovestin or Dienoestrol cream, 1 to 2 applicators full, two to three times a week; or Vagifem, 1 tablet twice weekly.

Helpful addresses

Menopause advice is generally available from family doctors, community health centres, family planning clinics, women's information centres and regional women's health education offices (via state health departments). Centres that specialise in menopause management include the following.

New South Wales

Centre for the Management of the Menopause, Paddington	(02) 339 4484
Family Planning Association, Ashfield	(02) 716 6099
King George V Memorial Hospital, Camperdown	(02) 516 7101
Nepean Hospital, Penrith	(047) 24 2167
Royal North Shore Hospital, St Leonards	(02) 438 7686
St George Hospital, Kogarah	(02) 350 2162
Westmead Hospital, Westmead	(02) 633 6333

Victoria

Baker Medical Research Institute, Prahran	(03) 522 4333
Family Planning Association, Richmond	(03) 429 1177
Jean Hailes Menopause Centre, Clayton	(03) 562 7555
Menopause Clinic, Monash Medical Centre, Clayton	(03) 550 2443

Menopause Clinic, Royal Women's Hospital, Carlton	(03) 344 2000
Mercy Hospital for Women, East Melbourne	(03) 270 2277
The Melbourne Menopause Centre, South Yarra	(03) 826 9799
Wainer Clinic for Women, Richmond	(03) 427 0399

Queensland

Annerley Women's Health & Family Planning Centre, Annerley	(07) 892 1149
Currumbin Beach Women's Medical Centre, Currumbin	(075) 34 2566
Princess Alexandra Hospital, Woolloongabba	(07) 240 2111
The Lilian Cooper Centre, Spring Hill	(07) 832 1666
The Queensland Menopause Centre, Wickham Terrace	(07) 831 7208
The Royal Brisbane Hospital, Herston	(07) 253 8111

South Australia

Ashford Hospital Medical Centre, Ashford	(08) 297 1777
Menopause Clinic, North Adelaide and Port Adelaide	(08) 239 1988
Endocrine Bone & Menopause Centre, Norwood	(08) 364 3274
The Queen Elizabeth Hospital, Woodville	(08) 345 0222
Queen Victoria Hospital, Rose Park	(08) 332 4888
Royal Adelaide Hospital, Adelaide	(08) 223 0230

Western Australia

King Edward Memorial Hospital, Subiaco	(09) 340 1355
Pivet Medical Centre, Leederville	(09) 382 1677
Women's Health Care House, Northbridge	(09) 227 8122

Tasmania

Family Planning Association, Cooee	(004) 31 7692
Family Planning Association, Devonport	(004) 24 7215
Family Planning Association, Launceston	(003) 31 9100
Family Planning Association, North Hobart	(002) 34 7200
Menopause Advisory Service, Hobart City	(002) 33 3508
Menopause Service, Launceston	(003) 37 2833
Women's Health Centre, North Hobart	(002) 31 3212

Australian Capital Territory

Family Planning Association, Canberra City	(06) 247 3077
Women's Health Service, Canberra City	(06) 205 1078

Northern Territory

NT Family Planning Association, Rapid Creek	(089) 48 0144

RESEARCH SOURCES

Armstrong, Bruce, 'Oestrogen therapy after the menopause – boon or bane?', *Medical Journal of Australia*, vol. 148, 7 March 1988, pp. 213–14.

Bachmann, G. A., 'Correlates of sexual desire in postmenopausal women', *Maturitas*, vol. 7, 1985, pp. 211–16.

Baker Medical Research Institute, *Annual Report*, 1992.

Bell, Glennys, 'The selling of HRT', *Bulletin*, 30 July 1991, pp. 38–43.

Burger, Henry (ed.), *Bailliere's Clinical Endocrinology and Metabolism: The Menopause*, vol. 7, no. 1, 1993.

Butler, Robert and Lewis, Myrna, *The Later Years*, Sun Books, Melbourne, 1986.

Cabot, Sandra, *Menopause: You can give it a miss*, Women's Health Advisory Service, NSW, 1991.

—— *Don't let your hormones ruin your life*, Women's Health Advisory Service, NSW, 1991.

Caplan, Gideon et al., 'The benefits of exercise in postmenopausal women', *Australian Journal of Public Health*, vol. 17, no. 1, March 1993, pp. 23–6.

Collins, Peter, 'Cardiovascular protection by oestrogen – a calcium antagonist effect?' *Lancet*, vol. 341, 15 May 1993, pp. 1264–5.

Coney, Sandra, *The Menopause Industry*, Spinifex Press, North Melbourne, 1993.

de Beauvoir, Simone, *The Coming of Age*, Putnams, New York, 1972, pp. 319, 346, 350.

Debelle, Penelope, 'The Keyte report', *Age Saturday Extra*, 1 May 1993.

Dennerstein, Lorraine et al., *Psychosocial and Mental Health Aspects of Women's Health*, Key Centre for Women's Health in Society, University of Melbourne, 1993.

—— 'Menopausal symptoms in Australian women', *Medical Journal of Australia*, vol. 159, 16 August 1993, pp. 232–6.

Dickinson, J. A. and Hill, A. M., 'The incidence of hysterectomy and its effect on the probability of developing uterine cancers', *Community Health Studies*, vol. xii, no. 2, 1988, pp. 176–81.

Diczfalusy, E., 'Characterization of the oestrogens in human semen', in Eckstein, P. and Zuckerman, S. (eds), *Memoirs of the Society for Endocrinology*, Cambridge University Press, no. 3, 1955, pp. 56–63.

Farrell, Elizabeth, 'Hormone replacement therapy – a rational approach', *Bioethics News*, October 1992, vol. 1, no. 1, pp. 25–34.

Finkel, Elizabeth, 'The great hormone balancing act', *Age*, 21 April 1993.

Fiske, Majorie, *Middle Age: The Prime of Life?* Thomas Nelson, Melbourne, 1979.

Ginsburg, Jean, 'What determines the age at the menopause?', *British Medical Journal*, vol. 302, 1 June 1991, pp. 1288–9.

Greer, Germaine, *The Change*, Hamish Hamilton, London, 1991, pp. 350–1.

Goldman, Lee and Tosteson, Anna, 'Uncertainty about postmenopausal estrogen', *New England Journal of Medicine*, 12 September 1991, pp. 800–2.

Jacobowitz, Ruth, *150 Most-asked Questions about Menopause*, Hearst Books, New York, 1993.

Jacobs, H. S. and Loeffler, F. E., 'Postmenopausal hormone replacement therapy', *British Medical Journal*, vol. 305, 5 December, 1992, pp. 1403–8.

Jennings, Garry (ed.), *Your Heart*, Text Publishing, Melbourne, 1992.

Khaw, Kay-Tee (ed.), *British Medical Bulletin Expert Review of Hormone Replacement Therapy*, vol. 48, no. 2, 1992.

Kiel, Douglas et al., 'Smoking eliminates the protective effect of oral oestrogens on the risk of hip fracture among women', *Annals of Internal Medicine*, vol. 16, no. 9, 1 May 1992, pp. 716–21.

Kingston, Margo and Date, Margot, 'Sterilisation takes over from the pill', *Age*, 20 January 1993.

Klein, Renate, 'The unethics of hormone replacement therapy', *Bioethics News*, vol. 11, no. 3, April 1992, pp. 24–37.

Llewellyn-Jones, Derek, 'The menopause', *Modern Medicine of Australia*, February 1984, pp. 32–3.

Lock, Margaret, 'Contested meanings of the menopause', *Lancet*, vol. 337, 25 May 1991, pp. 1270–2.

McCrea, Frances and Markle, Gerald, 'The estrogen replacement controversy in the USA and UK: different answers to the same

question?', *Social Studies of Science*, vol. 14, 1984, pp. 1–26.//
McKinlay, Sonja, *Women and Their Health in Massachusetts*, New England Research Institute Inc., Watertown, Mass., Final Report, 1991.//
MacLennan, Alastair, 'Oestrogen and cyclical progestogen in postmenopausal hormone replacement therapy', *Medical Journal of Australia*, vol. 157, 3 August 1992, pp. 167–70.//
—— 'HRT Regimens for the Menopausal Woman', *Current Therapeutics*, March 1993, pp. 43–8.//
Manson, JoAnn et al., 'The primary prevention of myo-cardial infarction', *New England Journal of Medicine*, 21 May 1992, pp. 1406–16.//
Mortimer, Derek, 'Views change on senile osteoporosis', *Australian Doctor*, 1 May 1992.//
Need, Allan et al., 'How to treat osteoporosis', *Australian Doctor*, 14 February 1992.//
North, Kathryn and Davies, Llewelyn, 'Postexercise headache in menopausal women', *Lancet*, vol. 341, 10 April 1993, p. 972.//
'Oestrogen implants can cause problems', *Australian Doctor*, 14 May 1993.//
'Osteoporosis researchers dig up the past', *Australian Doctor*, 2 April 1993.//
Reddy, Muriel, 'Dumped for a younger woman', *Sunday Age*, 21 July 1991.//
'Regular sex is important for female health', *Australian Doctor*, 28 February 1992.//
'Relaxation eases heart stress', *Australian Doctor*, 14 May 1993.//
Royal Australian College of Obstetricians and Gynaecologists, 'Consensus statement on hormone replacement therapy and the menopause', *RACOG Bulletin*, August 1991, pp. 19–20.//
Sheehy, Gail, *The Silent Passage*, Random House, New York, 1991.//
Silberberg, Suzanne and Burger, Henry, 'Management of the menopause from an Australian perspective', *Modern Medicine of Australia*, May 1989, pp. 14–21.//
Snyder, Raymond et al., 'Safety of post-menopausal hormone replacement', *Australian and New Zealand Journal of Medicine*, vol. 22, 1992, pp. 507–9.//
Spender, Dale, 'Alive & Sweaty', *Sydney Morning Herald*, 14 April 1993.//
Stanton, Rosemary, *Eating for Peak Performance*, Allen & Unwin, Sydney, 1988.

Taor, Adam, 'Oestrogen implants can cause problems', *Australian Doctor*, 14 May 1993.
Vandenbroucke, Jan, 'Postmenopausal oestrogen and cardioprotection, *Lancet*, vol. 337, 6 April 1991, pp. 833–4.
Westmore, Ann, 'More research needed into women's health', *Australian Doctor*, 15 November 1991.
—— 'Exercise: women are losing heart', *Australian Doctor*, 25 September 1992.
—— 'Long-term HRT use questioned', *Australian Doctor*, 9 October 1992.
—— 'Improving women's health', *Australian Doctor*, 7 May 1993.
Wilson, Robert, *Understanding HRT and the Menopause*, Hodder & Stoughton, London, 1992.
Wren, Barry, 'Society, the menopause, and hormone replacement therapy', *Postgraduate Medicine*, 22 August 1990, pp. 9–14.
Williamson, Margaret, 'How to treat the menopause', *Australian Doctor*, 27 September 1991.
Youngs, David, 'Some misconceptions concerning the meno-pause', *Obstetrics & Gynaecology*, May 1990, pp. 881–3.
Ziel, Harry and Finkle, William, 'Association of estrone with the development of endometrial carcinoma', *American Journal of Obstetrics and Gynecology*, 134, pp. 735–40.

INDEX

abdominal cramps, *see* cramps
ablation, endometrial, 100, 105, 142
aches, generalised, 31
acne, 45, 61
acupuncture, hot flushes and, 122
adrenal glands, 23
  sex hormone production, 23, 29, 173, 174
aerobic exercise, 132
aerobics, 51, 126
ageing, attitudes to, 31, 71, 162–3
alcohol, 46
  osteoporosis and, 81, 153
  sleeplessness, 125
amenorrhoea, 47, 82, 146
American Geriatrics Society, 36
anabolic steroids, 85, 131
androgens, 23, 48, 173–4
Anemone pulsatilla, 126
angina, 90
anorexia nervosa, 82, 146, 153, 154
antidepressants, 82
antipsychotics, 82
anxiety, 126
  hot flushes and, 29
  HRT and, 90
  influences on, 34
arthritis, 82, 144
aspirin, 99–100, 134
asthma, 82, 146
atherosclerosis, 89, 132–3
  oestrogen and, 89
  smoking and, 132–3
Australian Medical Association, 117
Australian Menopause Society, 169, 136
Australian Psychological Society, 117

Bachmann, Gloria, 109
backache, 26, 45
Baker Medical Research Institute, 86
barrier contraception, 135–6
Bates, Glenn, 110, 113
Beauvoir, *see* de Beauvoir
benzodiazepines, 82
bias, HRT studies and, 92–5
bilateral salpingo-oophorectomy, 68, 82, 143
biofeedback, 122, 124
biopsy
  breast, 159
  endometrial, 48, 99, 105, 139
bladder problems, 24, 25, 26, 77
bleeding
  abnormal, 48, 98, 139
  absence of, 58, 59
  assessment, 48
  breakthrough, 45–7
  duration of, 31
  fibroids and, 100
  heavy, 14, 19, 25, 46, 55, 61, 100, 142
  HRT and, 55, 138, 143
  hysterectomy and, 19
  irregular, 14, 19, 20, 21–2, 25, 28, 46, 55, 59, 61, 62, 64; *see also* breakthrough bleeding
  prolonged, 19, 25, 46, 61, 100
  withdrawal, 45–7, 53, 140
  see also period
bloatedness, HRT and, 43, 45, 102
blood clot formation, 46, 50, 51
  aspirin and, 134
  exercise and, 132
  family history of, 88

HRT and, 43, 89, 143–4
menopause and, 94
oestrogen and, 49, 89
personal history of, 99–100, 143
Pill and, 23
spontaneous, 99, 143
vitamin E and, 124, 134
blood fat
  assessment of, 47, 157
  exercise and, 132
  high levels of, 23, 65
  oestrogen and, 89, 93
blood flow, 89
blood glucose, 101
blood pressure
  exercise and, 132, 128
  falls and, 82
  ginseng and, 123
  high, 50, 51, 88, 99–100
  HRT and, 42, 43, 47, 49, 144
  Pill and, 23
  treatment of, 88
  vitamin E and, 124
blood vessels
  disease of, Pill use and, 22–3
  exercise and, 132
  HRT and, 86–90
  nutrition and, 133–4
  sex hormones and, 24, 34, 41
  smoking and, 132–3
  spasm of, 90
body build
  HRT dose and, 145
  osteoporosis and, 81, 156
  sex hormone production and, 23, 24, 25
body weight, 47, 102–3, 154
bone, 129–32
  calcium and, 154
  density, 26, 44–5, 47, 50
  density measurement, 65, 78–81, 152–3, 157
  exercise and, 81, 82, 154
  loss, 78, 90
  pain, 85
  peak mass of, 26, 78, 153
  sex hormones and, 24, 34, 41, 80, 172

smoking and, 82, 154
strength, 26, 153–4
see also osteoporosis
bowel
  cancer, 150
  prolapse, 26
brain
  neurotransmitters, 70, 74
  sex hormone effect on, 24, 172
breakthrough bleeding, 62, 64
  HRT and, 45–7, 105–6, 107
breast
  abnormal cells, 101
  biopsy, 159
  cancer, 46, 59, 95–7, 107, 141, 151, 158–9, 167
    family history of, 95
    oestrogen dose and, 95
  cysts, 152
  examination, 47, 64, 96, 101
  fibroadenomas, 152
  lumps, 101, 151
  mammogram, 47, 64, 96, 101
  progestogen and, 96
  sex hormone effect on, 24, 41
  soreness, 14, 54, 165
  tenderness, 45, 58, 84, 102, 107
Brecher, Edward, 109

caffeine, 81, 125, 153
calcitonin, 131
calcium, 130–1
  bioavailability, 131
  HRT and, 79
  loss, 79
  osteoporosis and, 81, 82
  sleeplessness and, 125
  sources of, 130–1, 155
Caldicott, Helen, 162
calendar dial pack, 57
Calendula officinalis, 126
camomile tea, 125
cancer
  bowel, 150
  breast, 46, 59, 95–7, 107, 138, 141, 148, 158–9, 167
  chemotherapy, 17, 20

endometrial, 37, 45, 59, 60, 85, 92, 97–8, 107, 138, 139, 142, 159, 161, 167
  ovarian, 98
  radiotherapy, 20
cardiovascular disease, *see* heart disease and blood vessel disease
cervix, 24
  mucus production by, 25
  sex hormone effect on, 41
chemotherapy, 17, 20
Chinese angelica, 134
chloasma, 106, 151
cholesterol
  high levels of, 23, 47, 65, 88
  measurement of, 157
  menopause and, 94
  oestrogen and, 89
Cimicifuga racemosa, 123
clitoris, 27, 115
clonidine, 123, 125, 152
clots, *see* blood clot formation
coeliac disease, 81
coffee, *see* caffeine
collagen, 74, 79
combined cyclical therapy, 57–8, 62, 141, 143, 151
concentration, 25, 66–7, 70
continuous combined HRT, 58–9, 62, 141, 143, 151
contraception
  anxiety about, 111
  barrier methods, 22
  menopause and, 21–3, 61, 62
  Norplant, 22
  Pill, 22; *see also* Pill
  sterilisation, 22
cramps, abdominal, 14, 45
culture
  menopausal symptoms and, 30, 73
  sexual activity and, 109
curettage, 48, 99
cyclical progestogen, 57–8
cyproterone acetate, 61
cysts, ovarian, 18

daughters, bone strength, 33, 154
Davies, Llewelyn, 51–2
de Beauvoir, Simone, 113, 118
decision-making, 70, 164–6
dementia, 162
Dennerstein, Lorraine, 169
depression, 33
  exercise and, 127
  HRT and, 90, 139
  midlife and, 31, 138–9
  non-hormonal therapies, 129
DEXA, 80
diabetes, 88, 101, 128
Diane-35, 61
diathermy, 142
Diczfalusy, Egon, 30
Dixarit, 123
dizzy spells, 25, 125
  exercise and, 128
  patch therapy and, 51
dose
  of HRT, 43–4, 144, 147
  reduction, 43, 149
dowager's hump, 78
dual energy x-ray absorptiometry (DEXA), 80
dual photon absorptiometry, 80
Dupin, Amandine, 68
Dwyer, Judith, 87

Eden, John, 55
eggs (ova), 21, 23, 25, 172, 173, 174
endometriosis, 17, 46, 62
  HRT and, 101–2, 107, 150–1
  hysterectomy and, 142
  surgery for, 18
endometrium, 17, 44
  ablation of, 100, 105, 142
  abnormal, 48
  biopsy of, 48, 99, 105, 139
  cancer of, 37, 45, 59, 60, 85, 92, 142, 159, 161, 167
  hyperplasia of, 44–5, 53, 60
  polyps, 104
  protection of, 53, 58, 59
  sex hormone effect on, 41

energy
  ginseng and, 123
  HRT and, 48, 75
  lack of, 19, 25, 31, 67, 74–5, 123, 127–9
Estigyn, 42, 43, 61, 84, 152, 175
Estraderm, 42
ethinyl oestradiol, 42, 43, 61, 84, 152
etidronate, 131
evening primrose oil, 14, 102, 124, 126, 151
exercise, 13, 47, 120
  aerobic, 132
  heart and blood vessel health and, 88, 132
  menopausal symptoms and, 33, 124, 125, 126
  osteoporosis and, 82–3
  plan, 128–9
  weightbearing, 82, 130
  wellbeing and, 71, 127

fat, production of oestrogen by, 39
fibroids, 19, 46, 55, 59
  history of, 19, 100
  HRT and, 55, 100, 107, 141, 143
  hysterectomy and, 142
Finkle, William, 117
Fiske, Marjorie, 113
flashes, *see* hot flushes
fluid retention, *see* bloatedness
fluoride, 131
flushes, *see* hot flushes
follicle stimulating hormone (FSH), 123, 172–3, 174
forgetfulness, 13, 14, 25, 70
  HRT and, 90
formication, 74
fracture, 46, 47, 78, 90
  HRT and, 38, 50
  risk of, 26
frequency, *see* urinary frequency
French paradox, 133–4

gall bladder disease, 101, 107
genetics
  menopausal symptoms and, 30

oestrogen levels and, 30
osteoporosis and, 82, 156–7
ginseng, 123, 124, 134
Greenblatt, Robert, 36
Greer, Germaine, 72, 73, 114, 117

hair, 61, 74
Hathorn, Libby, 110, 113
headache, 25, 31, 46, 122, 124–5
  HRT and, 51, 103, 144
  tension-type, 74
  see also migraine
heart, 24, 172
  disease, 15, 46, 51, 87
    family history of, 23, 88
    French paradox, 133–4
    HRT and, 23, 38, 65, 86–90
    in men, 158
    Pill use and, 22–3
    progestogens and, 89, 148
    risk factors for, 88, 156–8
    uncertainties, 89, 92–5
  exercise and, 128, 132
  nutrition and, 133–4
  oestrogen's effect on, 41, 172
  palpitations, 25
  smoking and, 132–3
heel bone ultrasound, 80
Henderson, Sara, 120
herbal treatments, 120, 123, 125
high blood pressure, *see* blood pressure
homeopathy, 120
hormone, *see* sex hormone
hormone replacement therapy (HRT)
  benefits, 66–90
  bleeding and, 45–7
  dosages, 43–4, 62–3, 175
  history of, 35–7
  options, 41–65
  risks, 64, 91–107
  types, 42
  user groups, 38–41
  ways of taking, 49–56
hot flushes, 12, 25, 46, 55, 66–70, 136–8, 172
  duration of, 27
  cause of, 12, 136–7

HRT and, 69–70
incidence, 24, 67
influences on, 29–30, 68, 137
non-hormonal treatments for, 122–4
placebo response and, 70
progestogen and, 61
severity, 11, 14
sleeplessness and, 11, 13, 30, 137
hyperplasia, endometrial, 53, 60
hysterectomy, 82
 bilateral salpingo-oophorectomy, 82, 143
 heart disease and, 88, 156, 157
 hot flushes and, 68
 implant therapy and, 55
 oestrogen and, 144
 osteoporosis and, 78, 79
 progestogen after, 141
 total, 18, 142–3
  incidence of, 18, 19, 142
  menopause and, 18
  reasons for, 19, 26
hysteroscopy, 19, 48, 99, 104, 105, 106, 139, 143, 159

implant, hormone, 29, 53–6
 rejection of, 56
 tachyphylaxis, 56
Inderal, 123
inhibin, 161, 172, 174
injection, hormone, 56
insomnia, *see* sleeplessness
insulin, 101
intercourse, 67, 76, 90, 141–2
 after menopause, 29
 painful, 18, 25, 29
International Menopause Society Congress, 141
irritability, 24, 25, 31, 58, 67
 HRT and, 106
 influences on, 34

Japanese women, attitudes to menopause, 30–1
joints, 24, 26, 31, 74
 oestrogen's effect on, 41

Karolinska Institute, 30
Kegel exercises, 126–7
Key Centre for Women's Health in Society, 169
Kinsey, Alfred, 109
Kostakidis, Mary, 163
K-Y jelly, 115

lactase deficiency, 130
laser, 142
lead, mood changes and, 73
libido, 24, 30, 61, 116–17
 HRT and, 41, 48, 90, 118, 139
 increased, 27
 loss of, 25, 27, 67, 75–7
ligaments, 74
lime blossom, 123, 134
linseed oil, 151
liver, 24, 47, 98–9
 HRT and, 43, 146
 oestrogen and, 41
Llewellyn-Jones, Derek, 24
lubrication, vaginal, 115–16, 141–2
luteinising hormone, 29, 137, 173

male dew, 30, 115
male, sexual activity, 109, 115, 118, 119
 bone density, 26
mammogram, 47, 65, 96, 101
marigolds, 126
Massachusetts Women's Midlife Health Study, 31, 38
mastectomy, 97
masturbation, 115–16
Medicare, 153
meditation, 122
Melbourne Women's Midlife Health Study, 31, 67, 70–1, 75, 103, 109, 124, 130, 132
memory lapses, *see* forgetfulness
menopause, 11–34, 135–6
 age at, 17, 20, 21, 135
 artificial, 17–18
 attitudes to, 16, 30–4, 163
 bone strength after, 26, 78
 contraception at, 21–3, 135–6
 definitions of, 16–17

early, 17–21, 78, 160
  experience of, 39–40
  influences on, 20, 21
  natural, 17, 21
  studies of, 32
menstrual periods, *see* periods
migraines, 31, 74
  treatments for, 103, 124, 125
mood changes, 24, 25, 33, 45, 72–4
  HRT and, 73–4, 90, 106
motherwort, 123, 134
muscle, 26, 74, 77
oestrogen production by, 39

naproxen (Naprosyn), 123
National Health and Medical Research Council, 87
National Women's Health Program, 32
naturopathy, 120
nausea, 50, 68
  HRT and, 51, 102, 107
nerve function, HRT and, 76
neurotransmitters, 70, 74
night sweats, *see* sweats
nipples, 27, 115
Norplant, 22
North, Kathryn, 51–2
Novak, Emil, 138
nutrition, 13, 46
  heart disease and, 88, 157
  menopausal symptoms and, 30, 33
  oestrogen levels and, 30
  osteoporosis and, 81, 153, 157

oatstraw, 126
oestradiol, 29, 41, 42, 171, 172
oestriol, 41, 172
oestrogen, 23, 30, 33, 39, 44
  conjugated equine, 36
  effects of, 41, 44, 69, 73–4, 77,
  heart disease and, 86–90
  hot flushes and, 29
  HRT, 34, 37, 41–3, 48, 49, 60, 61
  oestradiol, 29, 41, 42, 171, 172
  oestriol, 41, 172
  oestrone, 35, 41, 171

osteoporosis and, 79–86
requirements after menopause, 39–40
semen and, 30
smoking and, 84
tissues affected by, 24
uncertainties about, 93
vaginal preparations, 115, 118
Ogen, 42, 84, 175
orgasms, 76, 110, 114
osteoporosis, 15, 26, 46, 47, 77
  calcium absorption and, 131
  established, 85–6
  HRT and, 65, 77–86
  influences on, 81–4
  prevention of, 154–5
  risk factors for, 81–2, 156–7
  smoking and, 84
ova, *see* eggs
ovaries, 16, 17, 18, 22, 23, 24, 27, 168
  cancer of, 98
  cysts in, 18
  damage to, 17, 35
  osteoporosis and, 79
  removal of, 17, 18, 79, 143
overweight, 88, 132
ovulation, 21, 25, 172, 173
Oxford University, 73

palpitations, 25, 68, 74, 123–4
Panax herbs, 123
panic attacks, 126
Parker, Dorothy, 108
Pap smear, 47
patch, HRT, 14, 50–2, 106, 146–7, 150
peak bone mass, 26, 78, 153
Peck, Nancy, 32–3
pelvic floor muscles, 77
  exercises, 126–7
  prolapse, 26
perimenopause, 17
period, menstrual, 14, 16, 18, 33, 44
  heavy, 19, 25, 61
  irregular, 18, 19, 20, 21–2, 25, 28, 61
  prolonged, 18, 19, 25, 61
phyto-oestrogens, 129

Picot, Genevieve, 162
Pill, 42, 49, 61
  menopause, 22–3
  problems with, 43, 46
pills, HRT, 49–50, 146, 147, 149
plants, oestrogen-containing, 129
placebo, 70, 71, 75, 93
pre-eclampsia, 146
pregnancy, 21, 111
Premarin, 36, 42, 57, 175, 176
  blood pressure and, 144
  osteoporosis and, 84
premenstrual syndrome (PMS), 45, 47, 58
  hot flushes and, 68
  HRT and, 106
progesterone, 44, 173
progestogen, 19, 37, 44, 176
  effects of, 45
  HRT, 42, 57–8, 61
  osteoporosis and, 79
  progestogen-like substance, 61
  uncertainties about, 92
Progynova, 42, 84, 175
prolapse, 26, 127
propanolol, 123
Provera, 57, 58, 148, 159, 176
psychiatric illness, 71, 72
psychological symptoms at menopause, 70–2

quantitative CT scan, 80
Quit programs, 129

radiotherapy, 20
relaxation training, 122, 125, 152
Replens, 115
rheumatoid arthritis, HRT and, 144
rings, oestrogen-containing, 53
Royal Prince Alfred Hospital, 51

sadness, 67, 70
salt, osteoporosis and, 81
Sand, George, 68
sedatives, hot flushes and, 123
self-esteem, 26, 34, 70, 90, 118, 119
semen, as source of oestrogen, 30

sex, *see* intercourse
sex hormones 171–4
  fluxing, 26, 27, 28, 31, 68, 73
  influence of, 24
  measurements, 28–9
  production, 23, 30–1, 33, 38–9, 168
  receptors, 24
sexual activity, 29, 67, 75–7, 109–12
  male, 76
sexual arousal, 29
sexual intercourse, *see* intercourse
sexual interest, 67, 75–7
  male, 76, 117
  menopause and, 108–13
Shaw, George Bernard, 117
skin, 24
  chloasma, 106
  dry, 14, 74
  HRT and, 41, 106, 107, 147
  itchy, 74
  rash, 51, 106
  sensations, 25, 74, 115
  thin, 74, 147
  wrinkles, 74, 147
skin patch, 14, 50–2, 106, 146–7, 150
sleeplessness, 25, 67, 75, 109
  depression and, 139
  hot flushes and, 30
  HRT and, 90, 139
  non-hormonal treatments for, 125
smoking, 20, 23, 33, 46, 68
  benefits of quitting, 71, 128–9
  heart and blood vessels and, 88, 132–3, 157
  oestrogen and, 84
  osteoporosis and, 82, 131–2, 153, 157
Spender, Dale, 11, 24, 165–6
sterilisation
  female, 19, 22
  male, 22
steroids, 47, 146
  anabolic, 85, 131
  osteoporosis and, 81, 82
St John's wort, 126
stress, 13, 30
  hot flushes and, 30, 137

menopause and, 70–1, 73
sexual activity and, 109, 111
stroke, 23, 46, 86, 88, 134
sweats, 25, 66–70, 75, 109, 137, 165, 172
  after menopause, 31
  ginseng and, 123
  relief from, 90

tablets, HRT, 49–50, 146, 147, 149
tachyphylaxis, 56
tea, 125
temperature, hot flush rise in, 68
tension, 31
testosterone, 23, 24, 48, 61, 174
  libido and, 61, 77, 118
  HRT and, 48, 61, 62
thiazide, 131
thyroid disorders, 30, 146
tranquillisers, 67, 123
transdermal, *see* skin patch
triglyceride, *see* blood fat
Trisequens, 42, 175, 176
Tryptanol, 82
tubal ligation, *see* sterilisation, female

ultrasound, heel bone, 80
University of Melbourne, 169
University of New South Wales, 55
urethra, 24, 41, 77
urgency, 77
urinary
  frequency, 25, 26, 29, 52, 60, 67, 77, 90
  incontinence, 126
  tract infections, 25, 52, 60, 67
US National Institute of Mental Health, 139
uterus, 24
  lining of, *see* endometrium
  prolapse of, 26

vagina, 24
  dry, 14, 24, 25, 29, 46, 60, 67, 76, 90, 126, 141, 150
  examination of, 47
  infection of, 126
  lubrication of, 29, 52–3, 103, 115–16
  oestrogen and, 30, 41, 52–3
  thin, 76–7
  undiagnosed bleeding from, 99
valerian root, 125
Valium, 82
vitamins, 33, 124
  A, 126
  B, 14
  D, 131, 154, 155
  E, 14, 124, 134, 152
vomiting, 50
vulva, 24, 41

weight
  gain, 25
  HRT and, 102–3, 107
sex hormone production and, 23
wellbeing, HRT and, 72, 75
Wilson Foundation, 36
Wilson, Robert A., 36, 72–3
withdrawal bleed, 45–7, 53, 62, 104, 140
  absence of, 59, 105
  combined cyclical therapy and, 58, 103–4
  continuous combined HRT and, 59, 104
  fibroids and, 100, 104
  HRT and, 103–5
womb, *see* uterus
wrinkles, 74, 147

yoga, 122

Ziel, Harry, 117